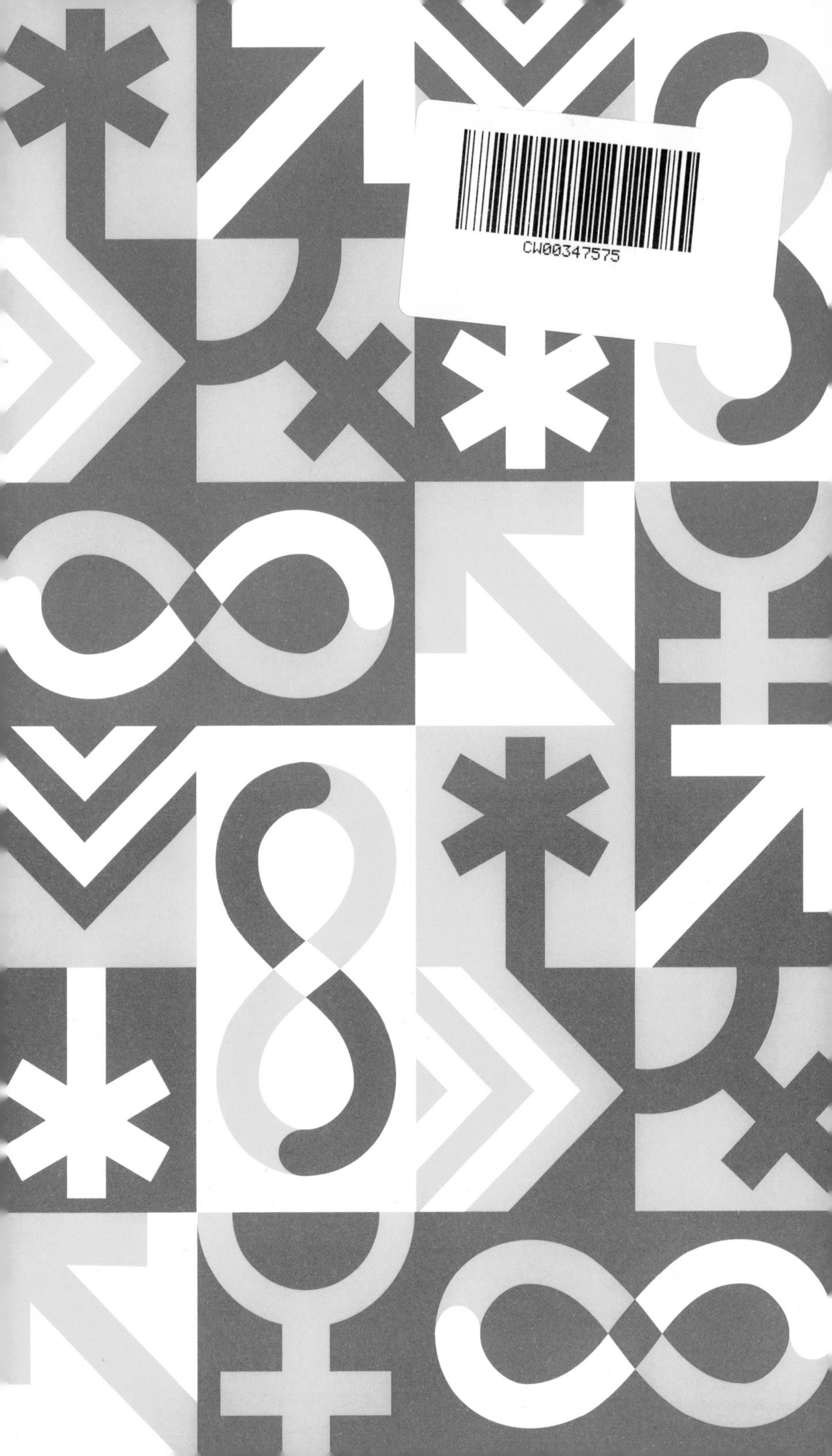
CW00347575

About the Authors

Carrie and David Grant have been regular fixtures on our television screens for decades. They were vocal coaches and judges on *Fame Academy*, judged the BAFTA award-winning *Glee Club* and have been part of several BBC primetime entertainment shows. Alongside co-authoring a bestselling vocal coaching book, Carrie has also contributed to various books on subjects such as mental health, child psychology and autism. Their broader services to society have also been recognised with MBEs: David for services to music and Carrie for services to music, media and charity. For the past ten years they have run a parent support group and Carrie has been involved in several campaigns and Parliamentary papers on the subjects of health and education.

Carrie &
David Grant

A Very Modern Family

Stories and guidance to nurture your relationships

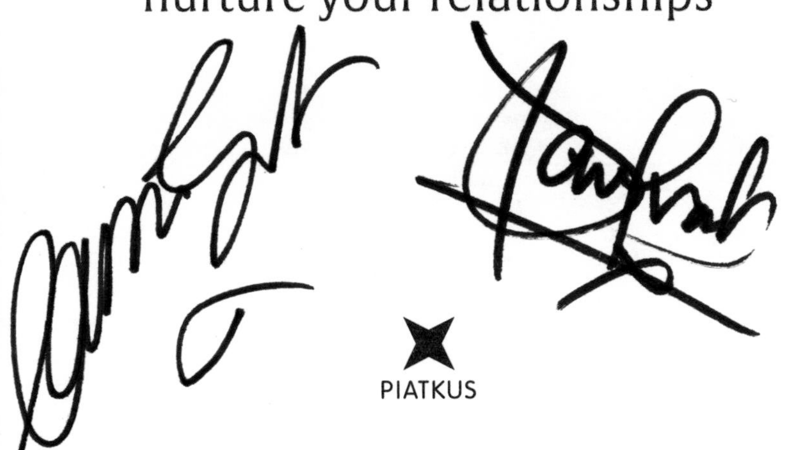

PIATKUS

PIATKUS

First published in Great Britain in 2023 by Piatkus

1 3 5 7 9 10 8 6 4 2

A CIP catalogue record for this book
is available from the British Library.

ISBN 978-0-349-43472-8

Typeset in Bembo by M Rules
Printed and bound in Great Britain by Clays Ltd, Elcograf S.p.A

Papers used by Piatkus are from well-managed forests
and other responsible sources.

Piatkus
An imprint of
Little, Brown Book Group
Carmelite House
50 Victoria Embankment
London EC4Y 0DZ

An Hachette UK Company
www.hachette.co.uk

www.littlebrown.co.uk

This book is dedicated to our four children,
whom we love without reservation.

You are our world and our inspiration.

CONTENTS

Note: Our first three children were assigned female at birth (AFAB). They had different birth names and back then their pronouns were she/her. In this book, in order to show the journey we have taken with this subject, we will initially use the genders they were assigned at birth but with their new names. Our children are Olive (they/them), Tylan (he/him), Arlo (he/they) and Nathan (he/him).

INTRODUCTION

It's spring 2009, and we have landed in Atlanta, Georgia. We are here to visit friends. David and I, plus our three children: Olive, aged fourteen, Tylan, aged seven, and Arlo, who is just two. We are a typical, happy family going on holiday, travelling on a shuttle train between the plane and the airport arrivals terminal. We are tired from the flight; the kids are a bit grouchy, but excited all the same. An announcement comes over the public address system, giving passengers directions about what to do once they depart from the train. When it finishes, the loudest feedback noise begins. It mildly disturbs the passengers; we exchange glances with one another, we eye-roll, everyone feels tired. Our three children all have their hands over their ears and look distressed. Our youngest, however, is experiencing something quite different, something outside the range of a normal response. Arlo has started to scream, so loudly, unceasingly, and at such a high pitch that the scream is giving the feedback noise a good run for its money. In fact, other passengers are beginning to be more affected by our screaming child than by the squealing PA.

Then, for the first time, the 'looks' begin.

I read their expressions. *What's wrong with that child? Why can't you control them? Do something.* David and I are down at our child's eye-level and, in an attempt to make Arlo hear us over their own screaming, we are trying to pull their hands off their ears, shushing them in a semi-empathetic, semi-authoritative, semi-panicked way. David picks them up, holds them, rocks them, comforts them. Nothing works.

We've tried everything within our current suite of parental skills, including giving Arlo 'the look', still the screaming continues. We've gently said, 'Enough now,' but Arlo is not listening. And then, as we exit the train, I give an assertive, emphatic and loudly whispered:

'STOP.'

'IT.'

Arlo is not having any of it. They scream for the next twenty minutes.

Airport terminals are never an easy experience for us. David being black means we are always on hyper-alert. It's a thing.

A real thing.

Almost everywhere we have gone over the years, we have written into our schedule the time allowed for the stop and search, the questioning, etc. A screaming child is not doing us any favours, drawing attention to us in ways we wish to avoid.

Eventually, we make our way through the terminal and to the relieving, welcoming faces of our friends. We relax and rest and chat endlessly, but over the next seven days, we realise something is not right with Arlo. Every noise, even the slightest sound, causes the same reaction as we saw on the shuttle train. The sound of doors slamming, the kettle boiling, or even the low hum of the fridge causes Arlo to put their hands over their ears in distress. Something's not right.

On our return to the UK, we made an appointment to see our local health visitor. She was one of those wise, sage, been-doing-this-for ever, empathetic kind of professionals that we have learned to treasure over the years, and would always long to meet. Arlo arrived in their off-the-shoulder attire, as was their custom with all clothes, played quite happily, talked about themselves in the third person – 'They want a drink. They want this toy.' – and then tried to undo the buttons of the health visitor's cardigan.

'I'm going to refer Arlo for an assessment. I think they may be autistic.'

Autistic.

Like many parents who've gone before us, this word didn't really mean much to us. On our return home, David and I did what we all do, and looked it up on the internet.

It wasn't a good read.

And we soon realised that the traits of autism we were reading about were also ticking a whole load of boxes for Tylan.

In the summer of 2009, David and I sit on the edge of a field in Berkhamsted and take in the news we've just been given. Two children with a certain diagnosis.

Two of our children are autistic.

As we watch them playing, our hearts are filled with joy and pain. Joy, because they are deliciously wonderful, creative and funny; and pain, because we realise the road ahead will not be as straightforward for our children as we had anticipated.

Autistic.

We have no idea what this means, good or bad. The label carries a weight we will all have to negotiate with.

Different.

Within minutes, we are talking about how different we ourselves are, and how varied people in the creative industries are, and how everybody loves the people who stand out in the world in which we work. The quirky are positively celebrated ... and in our very primitive, underinformed, uneducated but hopeful way, we begin the process of piecing together a new narrative.

The stories we tell ourselves about ourselves are shaped by many factors, but the underlying influence, our baseline for understanding who we are and how we relate to the world, is whatever we consider to be 'normal', and whether we match up to that standard, fall short of it, or stand outside of it.

Normal.

Steve Latham puts it this way: 'We consider to be "common sense" what is actually part of our culture. However, when anything appears natural or "neutral", then we know we are in the presence of a particular ideology.'[1]

Normal is the accepted wisdom; it's the majority. As we sit on the edge of that field, we face the prospect of once again being outsiders. We, who have spent our whole lives simply wanting to be regarded as equal to, or palatable to, those around us. The need to belong is hard-wired into each of us: some never have to think about it, some reject the concept, and others, like us, spend a large portion of their lives trying to join the party.

I think that day, we had a sense that things would have to change, that we would be drawn down unfamiliar pathways, that we would be reshaped by our experiences. Neither of us could have imagined just how much. What we didn't see was the fight we would have to endure for our children to be understood, for them to be heard and for their needs to be met. We didn't see the battles we would face on every front, grappling with inflexible systems outside the home, while trying to shape-shift in order to be the parents we needed to be inside the home. Nor could we have anticipated the division we would experience between us as we evolved into being all we needed to be for our children. We knew nothing of school refusal, self-harm, sitting by hospital beds on suicide watch praying for our child to live; we knew nothing of child-on-parent violence or gender dysphoria.

We knew nothing of the judgement,

or the exclusion,

or the isolation.

We also knew nothing of the absolute joy that would be felt when one of our children achieved even the smallest win. We knew nothing of the wild imagination of the neurodivergent brain or the wonder of their worldview. We couldn't imagine the sheer expanse of their creativity or the freedom that comes from living outside of the expected normative constraints. We didn't know about the exquisite belly-laugh-inducing family moments, nor the tears we would share with people who had walked through life alongside us and simply got it. We had no concept of the incredible family identity that would emerge, nor of how the power of love, tempered in the fire of challenge, would glue us together.

This would all come later.

The story that we will unveil in this book is one we have chosen to tell with our family's permission. Our story is their story – and may be, in part, your own story as you read this. The story is precious, and we ask that you hold it with respect. We are all still learning, we are growing and evolving, and we have chosen to tell it at this time because so many of the intersections being discussed in society right now are held within our family. For many years, we have been gatherers of people, networkers of different marginalised communities. Our home is rather like a community centre; people come for a cuppa and stay for a year! Our lives celebrate the individual in all their uniqueness, while placing the individual in the context of family and community. We need one another.

We are also rule-breakers. If any of us want to see change, the sentence we most need to hear or develop within ourselves is: 'We don't normally do it like this, but . . .' Rule-breakers will step into the unknown, break through hatred, fight for the other, stand up to injustice and face down giants. They are the people who have the imagination to dream of a better experience and a kinder, more diverse, more equal and inclusive world.

In writing this book, we have taken subjects we feel are key to our lives and growth, and it is our aim to show how we've managed to find the magic and make life work. You don't have to align with everything we have chosen to do, or agree with the way we think, but we do hope our thinking will challenge you to re-evaluate what you think about your own life and your personal situation. The idea is that we create the space for thought, for contemplation and for transformation.

As the stories unfold, we will take you back to different parts of our lives, covering the subjects we are talking about, and we will share the different experiences we have faced with our incredible children, how we've adapted, and what has really led us to our current outlook. You may also hear the voices of our children from time to time as they share their thoughts, and we take time to hear their voices.

1

Jumping Off

Change is inevitable. Change will ambush us at the most unexpected moments, swinging a wrecking ball that demolishes our preconceptions and lays waste to our current reality. Regardless of whether we accommodate and embrace it, or stubbornly resist it, change will happen. Whether it floors us or elevates us, our attitude to change is often shaped by our initial introduction to it. Some of us may remain mildly ambivalent, others of us will dream of it, chase it, crave it. And for some, it is the monster under the bed, that which must not be named, a threat to our very existence.

DAVID

Having children will change your life. Everybody knows that.

Father, Daddy, Dad.

Between Carrie and I meeting and the arrival of child number one, Olive, there were eight years. Three thousand, one hundred and fifty-three days, to be exact. If every day represents a learning opportunity, then I needed every one of those days. I had no clue about what being a father entailed. It took a further seven years before I was ready to have our second child, Tylan ... clearly, I was a slow learner.

This word 'father' is shot through with expectation, responsibility and threat. 'Father' is consistent, dependable, reliable, unwavering; it denotes security, solidity and certainty. Having never experienced 'father' myself, I was left feeling unable to bear the enormity of this unfamiliar title. I simply didn't believe I was equal to the task.

I'd only just got my head around being a husband, as I had never witnessed one of those at close range, either. Having been raised by my mother and grandmother, I feared I would be like my own father.

Absent.

Maybe I wasn't temperamentally predisposed to fathering. I was afraid that if there was an approved style of fathering, I didn't know it. I had so many fears, because I had so many unresolved father issues.

Carrie was six months pregnant, and I was sitting on the stairs in our flat, with the phone in my hand, willing myself to call my father. I had his number; he was living in America.

Sometimes, it's easier to feel negatively about a perceived enemy than to contend with a living, breathing, nuanced, real person.

There was still that part of me that was the seven-year-old standing on a Southampton dock, waving my father off on his journey back to Jamaica. He had entered my life like a whirlwind, two weeks earlier, and had promised to return in six weeks.

He never came back.

I waited thirty-one years for a proper conversation.

Now, as I sat by the phone, I was not interested in my fantasy world being demolished by exposure to reality. For thirty-one years, in the safety of my made-up world, Daddy was a baddy, and I was happy to leave him there. But now I had a serious problem. The toxicity that I had ascribed to the word 'father' had left me totally ill-equipped for the task of being a father in my own life. I knew the act of making this call would take down an ancient wall. I dialled his number over and over, and kept putting down the receiver before it rang. And then, finally, I found the courage.

'Hello,' said the voice.

'Hi, Dad, this is David.'

'Aah, David,' came a warm and loving reply.

The affectionate tone of his response caught me off guard; it was not what I was expecting. We spoke at length. I was awkward and somewhat cold, but he held the space for me to find my feet. I asked questions that had been decades in the making, finding myself way off script. He answered honestly and candidly. He made no excuses.

He spoke of the wrong he had done to me. He spoke of regrets and his efforts to put things right. He had sent many letters during my childhood. They were passed on to my mum, but in an act of loving protection, I had never received them.

But here he was, now, in the present, on the phone. He spoke of his life, and it sounded much like mine (minus his eight children). He wasn't perfect, but he was a world away from the 'Daddy the baddy' I had created in my head.

We cried together, we related, we connected.

These kinds of conversations don't always work out, but when both parties make way for love and reconciliation, it is the sweetest of experiences. My father's love, humility and acceptance of responsibility made it possible for me to extend clemency to him. He didn't ask for understanding, but I understood. He asked for forgiveness, and I forgave.

By the time I got off the phone, my defences had been well and truly taken down. Now I could begin to take the first steps into my fathering future. It would be a long road, and I still had a lot to let go of, but being shown love and exercising forgiveness had enabled me to begin the journey and provided me with a priceless key. As a father, as a parent, I would screw up. There is no such thing as a perfect parent. We are simply humans, trying to do whatever we can to make sure our children know we love them and that we are here for them; trying to prepare them as best we can to face the world and take their place in society with a sense of wholeness and purpose. In reconnecting with my father, I had just experienced the healing balm of having someone say to me, 'It wasn't your fault. I was wrong, I'm sorry.'

I was determined that my child would never have to wait a lifetime to hear those words.

CARRIE

Mother . . . Mum, Mumma, Mummy.

I play with the word in my head as I watch my belly move, the feet and elbows of the little and very wriggly person within. David and I have been married for six years, together for eight; we are so happy. Marriage works for us. I'm not sure how, but we seem to have cracked it.

A child.

What is this going to mean? Loss of our 'us'? Loss of freedom? An expectation that I should be a stay-at-home mum? When I was growing up, our motto was, 'Working-class people work,' so there's never been any chance of me being a stay-at-home mum, but inner expectations and the pressure I put on myself are overwhelming. My own single mum struggled so much, and over the years I've probably judged her parenting. Now I'll be under the microscope. I'll be judged.

What makes a good parent?

I have a sensation of being way off-piste, outside of my experience. I'm twenty-nine years old and I've never even held a baby before. Elif Shafak puts it perfectly in her book, *The Island of Missing Trees*: 'Worrying about how good a mother she would be to an unborn baby was like being homesick for a place she had not even visited yet.'[2] I really resonate with this when I think of myself back then.

On 3 December 1994 at about 10.30pm, Olive arrived.

A little girl: exactly what we had wanted.

Olive – not the name she was given at birth but one chosen later – was beautiful, with shiny, dark brown curls framing a stunning little light brown face. She looked around the room as if to say, 'Okaaaaay, so this is what goes on out here.'

Did I love her immediately? I'm not sure what love means in this context. I felt something so deep it went beyond love. She was a part of me, and as she stared intently into my eyes, it was as if we had always known one another. It was the same feeling I'd had when I first locked eyes with David eight years before. Somehow, my past and my future were right here, in the present, in this moment. I loved every part of

Olive. I loved every move she made, every noise she uttered, everything about her. I vowed I would never let anything or anyone harm her, that I would encourage her to live her best life and help her to achieve all her dreams. David and I spent those early days singing to her, making up new songs, dancing around the room, producing extravagant shows. Our home was filled with joy and an exquisite love.

David and I had been hesitant about having children, because we were afraid that a child may change the 'us' we had come to cherish. Adding Olive had been a big risk, and it had worked, but the thought of having a second child also brought us fear. It took us years to think about another expansion. What we did not see but later realised was that, as our ability to trust increased, our own childhood fears of abandonment diminished, and our capacity to love expanded. In line with this came a desire to grow a bigger family.

Tylan – the name she would later adopt – was born in 2001, seven years after Olive.

Another little girl. We were made up.

We understood girls, and as both of us had grown up with women only, we were super-confident that we knew how to raise them. Tylan was very different from Olive. Shy and quiet, with an air of 'knowing' about her, like an ancient wisdom. When she looked at you, she stared into your soul. She was poised and certain about what she liked and disliked. She was funny, with a totally unique sense of humour. She looked up to her big sister in awe and wonder. Both children were unbelievably creative: painting, drawing, writing songs, dancing, acting, always putting on a show.

We were all delighted when, five years later in 2006, Arlo was born.

All girls – great!

Arlo – this, again, the name she would later choose – was hilarious from the off. She brought the older two closer and was the focus of their attention. She was completely adored; she was super-cute and had her own way of being. If she didn't want to be sociable, she would simply not talk and block out any attempt at communication. If she wanted to socialise, she would walk straight into the middle of every conversation and demand attention. Looking back, and knowing what we know now, it makes sense, as Arlo is both autistic and has ADHD (attention deficit hyperactivity disorder).

And our love just kept on growing. I had babies in my twenties, thirties and forties, but we weren't finished yet. In 2011, a foster-carer friend approached me. She told me she was fostering her seventy-ninth child, a little mixed-race boy, who was about to turn two. This was significant, as those three factors combined – race, gender and age – meant he was less likely to be picked up for adoption. Would we consider adopting him? She passed me a photograph. A beautiful little boy in a pram that looked familiar; it was identical to the one we had bought back in '94 when Olive was born. All three children had used that pram, and when I finished with it, I passed it along. And along it went . . . through a number of different homes, until, years later, unbeknown to us, it landed at the foster-carer's house. The next picture showed him in a cot. The very same cot our children had all slept in. It was surreal. Could he be the final addition to our family?

Nathan.

The sweetest, loveliest little boy.

If we speak of love, then Nathan was always loved. Even from birth, he was never not loved. We protect Nathan's early life story, but what we will say is that not all parents are ready for the job of parenting, and being a parent to a new-born baby when you don't yet have the maturity, skills or resources is hard. If at the point your child arrives you are too broken to know what to do, there is a chance a baby will be neglected, even if they are loved.

Nathan had arrived at the home of my foster-carer friend when he was very young.

What should we do? How did we feel about adoption at this stage in our lives?

We took a very open-minded approach as we chatted it through with one another, talking way into the night, and we also discussed the concept of an addition to our family with each of our other children. David and I had resolved that the decision had to be unanimous. Every child categorically said, 'Yes.'

So, we said yes. It just felt right.

Six months later, Nathan walked into our family.

The ensuing years have been both exhilarating and challenging, sometimes impossibly so, but love has held this little family through all kinds of difficulties and change. Love has sustained us and kept us holding on when things have really pushed us. Love has led us into making tough decisions, defending our family's rights and fighting for survival. Love has driven us, every step of the way, to forgive, to accept one another just as we are, and to discover more of our true identities.

What we are learning along the way

1. There will never be a perfect time to begin the parenting journey.
2. Parenthood is not about being good enough, it is about growing into the role.
3. Familial love has the power to heal and restore. Breaking the umbilical cord to our own parents may be necessary if we are to become all we need to become as parents ourselves.

Questions for the reader to consider

1. Knowing the way in which you were parented, how do/will you parent?
2. What influences the way in which you parent?
3. Is there anything you need to let go of in order to become ready for the next season of life?

2

Identity: Neurodivergence and Mental Health

CARRIE

In this chapter, we will look at brain differences. By that, we mean those who are neurodivergent. The word 'neurodiversity' covers all diversity, while the divergent part of 'neurodivergent' means different to the majority. We should hold the thought in our minds that majority does not mean *right*; it simply means majority. We will also look at mental health issues that may arise in our children. It's worth pointing out that many of the strategies we have taken up or developed for our children work for all children.

Who we believe we are, who others believe us to be and who we actually are can sometimes be three completely different identities or perspectives on the self. As vocal coaches, the study of personal identity has been one of the most absorbing and rewarding parts of our work. The notion that every person on this planet is unique, has something distinctive to offer and a story to tell, leads us on a beautiful journey of discovery, as we dig, excavate, and uncover what lies beneath.

Of course, personal identity is drawn from several sources, including DNA, character, personality, culture, belief system and family set-up. It is also shaped by our life experiences, good and bad. For example, the way that David loves me changes me, transforms me and makes for a better me. Conversely, when I have suffered violence at the hands of my child, this invalidates me; it erases me and leaves me feeling monochrome. As we process different life events, we may get stuck, unable to move forward for a while, static in our concept of self. Once events have moved on, we may go back to being ourselves, but it's more likely that we incorporate what has occurred and another 'us' emerges. Identities never stop evolving, and, if we are curious, they never stop being worked on.

Each of our children has their own, very strong identity. Olive (they/them) holds a lot of opposites together: they are super-loud and yet often need to be quiet; they are very sociable but also need a lot of alone time. They are a connector of people. They are wise, very reflective and incredibly truthful and honest. They are talented at drama, music, writing, art, cooking. They are purposeful and determined. They have the heart of a campaigner. They are dreamy, spiritual and deeply interested in others.

Tylan (he/him) is empathetic and picks up on everyone's moods. He (as he is now) is kind and considerate, a loyal friend and a great listener. He is a gentle, strong and resilient fighter. He is talented at drama, music, art, martial arts and dance. He dreams big dreams and longs to make a difference in the world. He is also very spiritual.

Arlo (he/they) is hilarious! If Arlo is in the room, there is a constant cacophony of banter and back-chat. They are sociable and love having friends. They like being out and about, but also need lots of peace and quiet. They are talented at singing, playing instruments, art, cosplay and writing. They want to use their art, music or writing skills in their work. They are the person who is capable of delivering just the right one-liner at just the right moment . . . and equally capable of the exact opposite! They can be thoughtful and considered, and then in the next minute be impulsive and irrational. They are also a teen!

Nathan (he/him) is incredibly kind and helpful. He is the child who would do anything for you. He loves assisting people and is great at making friends. He is talented at anything to do with tech and is fascinated by how things work. He finds board games irresistible, and loves stats, figures and maths. He loves animals and currently dreams of being a farmer. He works well with his hands and loves to spend time happily alone in his own company.

These are small thumbnail sketches – overviews, if you like – of our children. They may also have other descriptors, but these are the features you would recognise if you spent any time with them. Yes, they may also have brown skin and be autistic or adopted or whatever; these are the headlines. Beyond these seen and unseen areas live the full identities of who our children truly are. As we grow and understand identity, there are always challenges along the way. Our senses of identity and self are shaped by our thinking, and so it follows that our mental health is of utmost importance. Sometimes we experience an onslaught on our thinking.

Mental Health

One thing the younger generation has understood well is the importance of looking after their mental health. The young have led the way with this; they are unashamed about tending to their mental health needs and have strategies for doing so. On the negative side, social media and reality TV have played a part in projecting the idea of the perfect life or perfect appearance – but mental health issues existed way before social media ever came along. The twitchy net curtains behind which a smorgasbord of family issues hide, and the gossip found in communities and small groups, have always existed.

Mental Health Check

In the younger generation, there is a definite drive to take the pressure off having to appear as if we have it 'all together'. Some in our society are starting to challenge the shame attached to not being perfect. This is good, but we still have an awfully long way to go. As parents, we want to get it right for our children regarding mental health; we don't want to overlook what might be happening right under our noses. So, what should we be aware of? We try to notice any obvious changes in our children, little clues, treating them like a breadcrumb trail that invites us to find them in the hurting place.

- We regularly check in with our children, creating an environment where it's normal to talk about feelings, fostering time and space where we share emotional news as well as day-to-day occurrences, where family chit-chat can easily slipstream into a 'Where's your head at?' conversation. Some people find it hard to talk about emotions, and so we may switch to talking about what they are experiencing physically. If our children cannot access feelings, sensations in the body can open up the conversation. We might ask things like, 'Does your body feel comfortable?' or 'Are you feeling that anywhere in your body?' If both emotions and sensations are difficult to draw out, then just asking for the hard facts – 'What happened today?' – can help.
- We try to be present with and 'read' our children. One child may withdraw at stressful times, another may present with behaviours that challenge us or their school community. It is normal for teens to want to spend time on their own in their bedrooms, so this is hard to look out for, but regular checking in can be helpful. They may tell us to go away, and sometimes we do, but, ultimately, the priority is that we are letting them know we are present and available.
- We notice general self-care changes, such as not washing or avoiding teeth brushing.
- We observe any eating issues, such as withdrawal from food, overstimulation with food, craving sugar, and so on.
- We also pay attention to changes in their sleep patterns. Anxious children often have trouble getting to

sleep; they may experience interrupted sleep or may want to stay in bed for long periods.

- Another area we take note of is any loss of enjoyment or enthusiasm for their out-of-school activities or social life. When a child disengages from their intense interests, we know we have a problem.

I recently interviewed therapist Natasha Ainley from Art Therapies for Children.[3] She works in schools across a number of boroughs in and around London. Natasha spoke about the children the organisation work with who experience challenges to their mental health. When I asked her about the youngest children they work with, I was shocked to hear they were working with children as young as four years old.

As of July 2021, one in six children aged five to sixteen were identified as having a probable mental health problem.[4] That is five children in every class of thirty. Nearly half of seventeen- to nineteen-year-olds with a diagnosable mental health disorder have self-harmed or attempted suicide at some point, rising to 52.7 per cent for young women.[5] YoungMinds reported that 80 per cent of children and young people they interviewed said that the Covid-19 pandemic was having a detrimental effect on their mental health.[6] In 2021, the NHS saw an 83 per cent increase in demand for urgent eating disorder services.[7]

These stats are frightening, but this is the landscape in which our children live. What can we do? With a lack of access to children's mental health services, we must work together to provide the help our children need. There is a greater emphasis on schools to make sure our children's mental health is protected and nurtured. It is essential that education, health and social care authorities and the family work together. In this way, we can bring change. Empowering children and parents is essential.

All too often, our services perceive parents and carers as a bother and our assets are overlooked. People who may have run companies, managed complex projects or organised all sorts of things in life are suddenly simply 'Mum' or 'Dad' – we don't even have our own names. Working together means trusting the strengths of the team, making everyone equal around the collaboration table. Parents and carers have incredible insight, and we need to make the most of this. We need to be able to come up with ideas, allowing good suggestions to come from anyone in the team. Everyone needs to agree on what to do – and then do it. We also need to be able to allow for failure. Fail forward – learn from the things that have not worked and be flexible enough to adjust the strategies.

We now appear to live in a society where the expectations of parenting have become polarised. Some parents bring massive pressure to bear when their struggling child is underachieving. The demands we make when our children are falling apart impact mental health. Equally, fussing over our children as though they are made of cotton wool disables them, as does helicopter parenting, where parents parachute to the rescue with every challenge. This does not build resilience in our children. Both extremes are unhelpful. Our children need balance, and they need us to be able to read them. To know when to push and when to pull, when to step in and when to back off. If our children have additional needs, we have to become incredibly sensitive to the 'push and pull'. With additional-needs parenting, we will spend a lot of time in between, simply holding the space and waiting patiently.

Practical Action

There are also practical things we can do. There is no doubt that social media has a part to play in both helping and hindering our children's mental health outcomes. Teaching our children to curate their social media is essential. Curating your social media is like choosing the books to go on your bookshelf. Making sure they access age-appropriate apps is important. Over the years, we have met many children who have had Facebook or Instagram accounts by the age of eight, when the access age is meant to be thirteen years old.

To prevent self-harm and death by suicide, we have all our medications in locked safes, and we hide all blades of any kind, including pencil sharpeners, shaving tools, etc. Of course, our children can access these things in other ways, but at least it sends out a message that we are 'holding the space' for mental health challenges and removing easy access to the temptations.

Like many other children who are different, our children have been bullied: in school, face to face and online. How do we create communities who love and accept one another? How do we go against the tidal wave of division? These are questions we all need to ponder, and we must work on the solutions together.

Our mental health is shaped by our concept of self and the circumstances and life events we find ourselves living with. Helping our children to develop a positive image and opinion of themselves is important, and leads to healthier self-talk and self-belief.

Labels

The composite parts of our identity can be drawn from many sources. But what about labels?

All our children have diagnoses of additional needs. Olive has ADHD (attention deficit hyperactivity disorder) and dyspraxia; Tylan is autistic and has dyscalculia; Arlo is autistic and has ADHD; and Nathan has ADHD, dyslexia and DMDD (disruptive mood dysregulation disorder). We will explain what all of these mean as we go along.

Everyone has an opinion on labels; some people are very strongly anti-label.

A label is only a problem if you have a problem with the label. A label is often the result of a hard-won fight for an assessment, leading to a diagnosis that may have taken years to come by. The fight for an assessment is usually driven by the need for an explanation of unusual or irregular behaviours that fall outside the expected norm. Seeking expert input and advice isn't wrong and shouldn't open parents up to malign accusations of trying to label their child. On the contrary, parents should be commended for making every effort to gain understanding. Knowledge is power, so none of us should be criticised for making an effort to empower ourselves with as detailed an understanding as possible of what we are witnessing and experiencing.

Once we have a rationale for why a child may behave the way they do, the onus is on everyone to make sure they know what that designation means. It is for the community around the child to be curious and interested, to regard each person as an individual rather than a type. If everyone truly knew and accepted what autism looks like in its myriad forms along the spectrum, there would probably be no need to have the label; people would just notice the traits and adapt accordingly. As it stands, people aren't aware, and this ignorance means autistic children and adults can have very negative experiences and feel like no one 'gets' them.

The neurodivergent community faces resistance. People say things like, 'We didn't have all these issues when we were kids.' This is both inaccurate and unhelpful. We *did* have all of these differences; we just sidelined, ignored, bullied or misdiagnosed these people – or locked them away.

Labels matter. When seen through a positive lens, labels become descriptions, explaining a person both to themself and others. But labels are not the sum total of a person, and it is important to look beyond labels, remembering we are complex human beings with many similarities and many differences. A label is a signpost to help you to understand.

When we were first trying to figure out our children, it was very confusing. We were completely ignorant about the different neurotypes. We thought that ADHD was those loud boys bouncing off walls, that autistic children were those who didn't speak or make eye contact, and that dyslexic people struggled to read and write. The truth is, these are incredibly narrow descriptors, bearing little or no resemblance to our children and the many like them.

Often, different neurotypes look different in males and females (i.e. those assigned female and those assigned male at birth), but there is also crossover. One of the issues we have had in the autism community is that early studies of autism were undertaken exclusively with boys – until relatively recently, it wasn't even believed that girls could be autistic, which would account for the high numbers of women in their forties and fifties now being diagnosed. The rates of autism diagnosis are increasing year on year. In fact, there was an exponential increase of 787% in recorded incidence of autism diagnoses between 1998 and 2018.[8]

ADHD

When Olive started school, we began to notice the differences between them and the other children. Olive had a shorter attention span, they were easily distracted, they fidgeted, they had intense interests, and they were clumsy and sometimes couldn't judge the physical space around them or the volume of their own voice, so would often speak loudly. There are many other traits for ADHD in girls (those assigned female at birth), including:

- an apparent lack of motivation
- forgetfulness
- being highly sensitive to noise
- talking a lot but not listening
- appearing withdrawn
- being easily upset
- being messy
- verbally impulsive; blurts thoughts and interrupts others
- showing poor time management

Of course, many of these could be seen as part of a child's development so it's vital to look at the whole picture.

You'll find a very useful full list of traits on the Verywell Mind website.[9]

Olive didn't tick all of the twenty traits listed, but they ticked a fair few. No one picked up on this in school. Unfortunately, the same is true for many children of colour. A disproportionate number of black and mixed-race children are sent down a Social Emotional Mental Health (SEMH) pathway rather than a Special Educational Needs (SEN) pathway.[10] In other words, some teachers are more likely to translate challenging behaviour as a social problem, issues within the home, rather than a brain-wiring issue. So, Olive was considered to be naughty. When they were distracted, it was read as defiance. When they clicked their pen incessantly, it was assumed to be blatant rudeness. No one looked deeper into what was actually happening for our child, and so we were none the wiser. They were eighteen years old by the time they were diagnosed. By then, they believed themselves to be both a bad person and academically and intellectually inferior to others, and it took a long while to come back from those overwhelming and erroneous feelings. If adults misjudge us when we are young, it's hard to believe they are wrong. At home, we positively celebrated Olive's ways of being and found them to be a compliant, curious and incredibly bright child, but at school it was a different story.

Autism

In some ways, it was the same for Tylan: no one noticed he was different and that he was struggling until he was much older.

TYLAN

I was diagnosed as autistic at the age of seven, but the school didn't believe the report to begin with, because they only had one view of what autism looked like and I didn't fit that mould. I just remember going into school and feeling like I was an alien. I knew I didn't fit in, and as much as I tried to, I just couldn't manage it. I would 'mask' all the time. Masking is where you try to blend, copy and pretend you are not super-anxious. I am very good at it, hence why being an actor is a good job for me. In school, I would somehow manage throughout the day, but inside I was melting down. I would wait till I got home from school and then let it all out. Melting down is not like a tantrum, which lasts maybe ten minutes and then burns out. A meltdown can last ninety minutes and leave me feeling completely exhausted. No one in my school understood me. It wasn't just the other children; it was also the teachers. I never felt safe or seen at school, and after a while I just refused to go any more. We were also told in school that our school days were the best days of our lives, and this led to feelings of real hopelessness and depression. If this was as good as it was going to get, then what was the point of living? There was nothing to look forward to; there was no hope. I was really shocked when I finally got to leave school at the age of sixteen, and discovered that the adult world was far kinder than my experience of school.

One day, a family friend, Georgia, told me she had seen an advert on Facebook. *Hollyoaks* were auditioning for an autistic person to play an autistic character. I would go on to become the first autistic person of colour playing an autistic character in a UK soap. Suddenly there was representation, and I was it. I had never seen anyone who was like me anywhere on TV, or in films, art, music or books. As a child, I longed to see people like me, and people who looked like me. If ever there was a case for needing more representation, this was it. Children need to be able to see themselves as they are growing up.

Leaving school was the best thing to happen to me. Before I arrived on set for the first time, Lime Pictures, who make *Hollyoaks*, sent every member of the cast and crew for autism training. To give you a sense of what that means, a lighting rigger on *Hollyoaks* has had more autism training than any teacher who ever taught me in my whole time in school. In that first year at work, I was nominated for various awards and that really meant a lot. For a child who felt totally unseen by the outside world, it felt good to be noticed and heard.

Getting a Diagnosis for Autism

CARRIE

The other thing about labels is that they come from (or should come from) having had an assessment and a formal diagnosis. Delays in diagnosis can be a real issue. As of March 2022, there were over 100,000 people in England alone waiting for an assessment for autism.[11] Often, children and adults wait years to find out what's happening within themselves. If schools are not trained to spot the many and varied presentations of a particular neurodivergence, children get missed. Those children grow up feeling as though they are stupid and that they don't fit in. It is not best practice to diagnose oneself and assessments should be sought, even if the waiting lists are long. Neurological conditions and life experiences, for instance trauma, can have traits that overlap, so it's important to know what you are dealing with.

We have been shocked by the waiting times. Waiting up to eight years for an assessment is not uncommon in the UK. Since we have started navigating 'gender', we have heard there are also waiting lists of thousands in this area; one parent recently told us their child was on a sixteen-year waiting list for an appointment at a gender identity clinic!

I have never met anyone who has been grateful for a late diagnosis. To find out you are autistic in your thirties, forties or older may produce an initial response of absolute relief, but it can also lead to long periods of grief and regret, mainly because people have spent their whole lives being told they are difficult, they are fussy, they are too much, or they are less than. Having a diagnosis explains you, both to yourself and to others.

Here are a few of the common traits of autism:

- taking things literally
- appearing insensitive
- seeking solitude
- difficulty forming friendships
- highly anxious
- a preference for routine

If you want to delve deeper into autism traits the National Autistic Society has a very good website with lots of information.

The last two points outlined above are important in terms

of the day-to-day challenges for autistic people. According to the National Autistic Society[12]:

> With its unwritten rules, the world can seem a very unpredictable and confusing place to autistic people. This is why they often prefer to have routines so that they know what is going to happen. They may want to travel the same way to and from school or work, wear the same clothes or eat exactly the same food for breakfast.
>
> Autistic people may also repeat movements such as hand flapping, rocking or the repetitive use of an object such as twirling a pen or opening and closing a door.

Because Tylan wasn't believed to be autistic, it led to invalidation in primary school and meant the necessary adjustments were not made for him until his final year in secondary school. He ticked every academic box, he looked like he had friends, and it was assumed he was managing in all areas of school life, like the canteen, the toilets and the playground. No one noticed how challenging school was for him. No one noticed he was being bullied for being different, and Tylan didn't have the words to explain that bullying; he just assumed this behaviour was how friendships worked and tried all the harder to fit in. No one noticed he was terrified by the black-and-white photographs used in history lessons, or the overwhelming feelings he was experiencing due the noise of the class or the smell of onions on the teacher's breath.

Some would say this was because Ty was 'under the radar' or 'high functioning'. High functioning is a horrible term, and not very fair if the person is finding it near-impossible to function in life. In our family, we call it neurotypical passing.

This feels like a truer descriptive, and shows the problem for many autistic people when society doesn't recognise their autism.

When Tylan moved into secondary school, we hoped things would change. Even though this school understood Ty was autistic, it made no real difference. Tylan's needs were not communicated thoroughly enough, and very few teachers understood how he was experiencing the world. Unfortunately, Tylan was blamed and shamed for being different – by children and teachers alike. Inside, he was immobilised with anxiety and fear, and every day was a minefield of challenges that meant going to school was like entering a war zone. I do not use that term lightly. In 2019, Callum Wetherill, pastoral leader of Joseph Norton Academy, said: 'We're getting a high influx of students coming in with high levels of institutional trauma, rather than lifelong developmental trauma.'[13] Many of our most vulnerable children are developing PTSD-like symptoms as a result of the trauma experienced in school.

Mental Health in Our Family

'Can you kill me, please?'

Those were the chilling words said to me by our ten-year-old, Tylan. The request was measured and calm.

I answered very clearly and definitely: 'No, I cannot do that for you.'

Hours later, as I lay in bed, I began to process the enormity of what was happening and my absolute and utter powerlessness to make a better world for our child. This situation would go on for years, right up until the day he left school, but in those first moments I knew I would have to assume a new identity.

A warrior parent.

Warrior parents are not born. My warrior parent identity was forged in the furnace of watching the affliction of my children. I would rage against the injustice. I saw our child suffer, paramedics being called, our child lying in a hospital bed, bullying messages coming on to their phone as they lay there, the bullies telling Tylan to kill himself, me saving his life while trying to access mental health services. If the education system had failed our child, the health system didn't fare much better.

A 2019 YoungMinds report showed that Children and Adolescent Mental Health Service (CAMHS) only accounts for 0.7 per cent of overall NHS spending,[14] and yet evidence shows 50 per cent of mental health issues begin by the age of fourteen.[15] In July 2021, I posted a tweet, having read a quote from our then-Minister of State for Mental Health, Suicide Prevention and Patient Safety, the Rt Hon. Nadine Dorries MP. At an all-party parliamentary meeting, Dorries said, 'CAMHS is well resourced and robust.' I simply added to the quote, 'Has anyone got anything to say about this? What's your experience?'[16]

That tweet, with its four million impressions, trended for two days. From mental health specialists to teachers, parents to doctors and children's mental health administrators, all told the same story of a service doing its very best while under-resourced, stretched to breaking point and barely scratching the surface of the avalanche of children's mental health needs. The Twitter responses told the painful, real-life experiences of forgotten people.

Prior to Covid-19, global figures for depression and anxiety, two of the most common mental health conditions of childhood, were estimated to be 8.5 per cent for depression and 11.6 per cent for anxiety. The latest meta-analysis suggests significantly higher rates for clinically significant depression (23.8 per cent) and anxiety (19 per cent) in children and adolescents, a more than two-fold increase in prevalence rates compared with those reported prior to the pandemic.[17]

What does this mean on the ground, where parents and children are tearing their hair out trying to get help? In 2017, I hosted NHS England's annual conference, where Clare Murdoch, director for mental health, talked about the 'Five Year Forward View for Mental Health'.[18] At the time, Murdoch shared that only 25 per cent of referrals to CAMHS led to an appointment. She promised this would change, and it has. We are currently five years on from that promise, and the figures don't paint a pretty picture. Even though there was an improvement of 4 per cent, post-pandemic, the referrals have risen by 39 per cent.[19] Put simply, parents can access little or no help for their children. Unfortunately, most children do not meet the threshold for an appointment. Parents are left to work things out for themselves, and they often find themselves wrung out, stressed and anxious about their child's future.

Obviously, there are many children who are not neurodivergent who have mental health issues, but the big question in the backs of our minds is always this: if the world was a kinder place, would our children's mental health be better, or are some of their mental health challenges a direct result of being neurodivergent? Deep down, we really feel that the former, not the latter is the issue.

Traits and Tropes

Understanding who we are, who we are becoming and the general complexity of ourselves takes a lifetime as we constantly shift and change. Grappling with our own evolving identity while trying to get a deeper comprehension of the children in our charge is doubly difficult. Children are on a constant journey of discovery, and are always pulling something new out of the bag. As a new part of each child emerges, we shape-shift around it.

There is a phrase that goes, 'If you've met one autistic person, you've met one autistic person,' and this is true.

Every autistic person is different, and the traits that occur in one person may be totally different to another, which is why it's important not to make tropes out of the community. Just as we have seen with other identities, such as culture, sexuality and gender, tropes are the most unhelpful descriptors, boxing people in with an expectation of behaviours and responses. Saying 'all autistic people are . . .' or 'all black people are . . .' or 'all gay people are . . .' does a disservice to those people.

Understanding the traits or areas that *may* arise from being autistic are helpful, and there are many times, even as we are writing this, that we have had to refer to clinical experts to discover a new area we hadn't heard about before. Here's one such example that happened recently.

David and the kids love watching *Stranger Things* on Netflix. Lots of people are mad about *Stranger Things*; it's a cult series. But one of our kids really loves *Stranger Things*. And when I say they love it, I mean they're literally obsessed! This is what's known in the neurodivergent world as a special interest. That is, an intense interest in something that goes beyond enjoyment or being a fan and becomes a lifestyle.

Over the years, our children have obsessed over so many things, including loom bands, *Glee*, *Frozen*, the Muppets, buttons, *Night in the Woods* and many, many more. A special interest means our children will want their entire world to reflect that interest. The interest is sometimes used helpfully in school to assist autistic children with engaging. It can also create a career path. The special interest often gives an autistic person a sense of safety or of being soothed.

But – back to *Stranger Things*.

Arlo loves *Stranger Things*.

Arlo particularly loves Eddie Munson from *Stranger Things*.

Arlo wants to dress like and look like Eddie Munson.

. . . Now Arlo thinks they *are* Eddie Munson from *Stranger Things*.

Now Arlo is talking as themselves to Eddie Munson and then answering as Eddie Munson.

Late at night, in crisis, they talk to us as Eddie Munson.

This thing has now, at certain times, taken over.

So, what's happening here?

David and I have been worried that perhaps Arlo is experiencing dissociative identity disorder (DID). Is it psychosis? Big words with big fear.

We spoke to our local mental health team, who told us they had noticed this experience can happen with autistic people. It can be a coping mechanism, especially when they have a lot of worry and their anxiety is raised.

Arlo is in the middle of GCSEs, and things have been very difficult recently with one of the other children. There's a lot going on, so they are especially anxious, and apparently this absorption into another character can be an anxiety response.

Now, that is a relief. Not because we can forget about it – we can't – but because we can work from a position of knowledge, understanding this has its roots in anxiety, not identity or another condition. We can do more to think about how to reduce anxiety for Arlo and give them extra attention where necessary.

Overlapping Traits

Overlapping traits are also something we don't really understand much about, and can be a reason for why people are sometimes misdiagnosed. The professionals are under huge pressure to keep up to date with the latest science and thinking, and they have to get it right.

People with ADHD, autism and DMDD will all experience issues with what is known as sensory integration. In layman's terms, at the base of the brain are two clusters of cells known as the amygdala. The job of the amygdala is to regulate emotions by processing the information received via the body's five senses. The amygdala processes this sensory information and judges if it is good, bad, or indifferent. This influences the decision-making part of the brain, with its fight, flight, freeze or fawn responses.

The amygdala of young autistic children can be smaller or enlarged,[20] and scans have shown the amygdala in people with ADHD can be smaller.[21] In our children, this gateway to processing sometimes takes in too much information and at other times not enough, and this can lead to increased anxiety, which in turn can lead to unwanted responses and impulsivity. In effect, all our children are experiencing the world in a super-sensitive way, and this leads to very high levels of anxiety.

Our children all have intense interests, social anxiety and some OCD-like traits; they are somewhat or totally demand-avoidant, and they may be more susceptible to dysphoria or eating issues, depression, self-harm and suicidal ideation. Trauma can also exacerbate these traits. With our two autistic children, there are issues with social communication that are vastly different, even to one another. They express and receive communication in different (not less-than) ways. With all of this going on, can you imagine how hard they have to fight to discover their identity?!

And, of course we can't ignore all the disses . . . dyslexia, dyscalculia, dyspraxia. Running alongside the other areas, some of our children also have these diagnoses. When children are assessed, they are diagnosed according to what is known as the DSM-5, the *Diagnostic and Statistical Manual for Mental Disorders.*[22] It's constantly updated, and all appropriate health professionals have to use it. To achieve greater accuracy for girls, women and those assigned female at birth going for an autism assessment, it is often recommended that in addition to the DSM-5 assessment tool, the Diagnostic Interview for Social and Communication Disorders (DISCO)[23] form is also used.

Dyslexia

Nathan is twelve years old and barely writes. He can write his name, but sentences are still a struggle for him. He reads better than he writes. Nathan has dyslexia-like traits, but reading and writing challenges can originate from a whole range of issues, including trauma. Nathan has a complicated and layered diagnosis, so is not typically dyslexic, but here are just some of the most common symptoms listed by the NHS:

- delayed speech development compared with other children of the same age (although this can have many different causes)
- problems expressing themselves using spoken language, such as being unable to remember the right word to use, or putting sentences together incorrectly
- difficulty with, or little interest in, learning letters of the alphabet
- spelling that's unpredictable and inconsistent
- confusion over letters that look similar and putting letters the wrong way round (such as writing 'b' instead of 'd')
- confusing the order of letters in words
- reading slowly or making errors when reading aloud

You'll find a more comprehensive list of the symptoms of dyslexia on the NHS website.[24]

Dyscalculia

Dyscalculia is a very similar condition to dyslexia, but whereas dyslexia concerns words, dyscalculia concerns numbers. Tylan has dyscalculia, and it is amazing how many different areas of life are impacted by this condition. Working out train times and how many minutes are left before he has to leave the house, telling the time and measuring things are all a challenge for him. The Dyslexia Association[25] website has a lot of information, including some on dyscalculia, as the two conditions are very similar. Here are just some of the common symptoms of dyscalculia:

- poor mental arithmetic skills
- has difficulty counting backwards
- still uses fingers to count
- struggles to understand mathematical symbols such as +, –, × or ÷
- has a tendency to put numbers in the wrong place or column
- finds it difficult to keep the score in games
- struggles to understand the meaning of charts and graphs

A full list of symptoms can be found on the Dyslexia Association website.[26]

Dyspraxia

Olive has dyspraxia. This is where someone struggles with motor skills. This could mean large motor skills, like balance and coordination, or fine motor skills, like writing. Olive was diagnosed at the age of eleven. There are some overlapping traits with ADHD, which is probably why it took a further seven years to diagnose their ADHD. Olive's dyspraxia shows in their fine motor skills, and as a young child it affected their handwriting the most. They would hold the pen tightly and write heavily. By the age of eleven, they had a reading age of eighteen, with a vast vocabulary, but writing was painstakingly slow. This was particularly difficult when it came to writing stories. Olive worked at super-speed, creating long, multi-level narratives with complicated plots, but they had only a frustratingly snail-paced ability to write these ideas down. From when they were about seven, I would record them and they would then write down what they had said. Sometimes it would take a whole hour to write one sentence. Inevitably, Olive would become impatient and refuse to continue, and then it felt like homework was just an exercise in disciplining my child. Sometimes, the homework session would go on for hours. I would be sending them to the naughty step for refusing to do the work.

To be honest, looking back, I really hated that our children had homework from such a young age. Even in reception, schoolwork would be sent home. Home was the place where they felt safe, away from the difficulties of school – but then school followed them home in the shape of homework. There is no evidence to show children do better in school for having done all this homework. Here are some of the symptoms of dyspraxia:

- struggles when playing with toys that involve good coordination
- difficulty with activities such as hopping, jumping, running and playing with a ball
- finds writing, drawing and using scissors challenging
- difficulty getting dressed, tying shoelaces and doing up buttons
- may have a poor attention span and find it difficult to focus on one thing
- may appear clumsy – often dropping or spilling things

- difficulty making friends
- behaviour problems – often stemming from frustration

There are many more symptoms and they can vary with age so it's worth seeking out more information if this rings any bells with you. The NHS website has a comprehensive list of symptoms.[27]

Even as Adults, Our Identities Are Evolving

Watching our children suffer changed my identity. It birthed a new me: a me who would care more than ever about changing systems, challenging the status quo and demanding improvement for our children and those like our children. It made me want to kick down metaphorical doors, to shout for access, to keep calling out unfairness and to negotiate the change that would make a difference for children like ours. I had always longed to be a change-maker, but I could never have imagined this would be my route in.

Even now, deep in my heart, I long for a time when children like ours will walk through open arches where locked doors once existed. As parents, we want to be the bridge each of our children needs us to be. The bridge that allows the transition between one world and another. We want to be good allies. When I watch those who are different from the cultural normative having to give a reason for their existence, it reminds me how important allyship is. We also encourage our children to advocate for themselves and for others. For us, it is an important part of raising our children to take their place in society.

I am super-aware that we only have a few years to get this stuff right. We only have a few years to make sure our children are world ready. Our job is to help them to understand themselves. We encourage them to explore their identity; we gently shepherd them towards making good choices.

When parents say, 'I just want my child to be happy,' I always feel this does a great disservice to our children by placing an impossible expectation on them. No one is constantly happy so it's a huge ask. We want our children to be able to navigate this world with all its challenges. We want them to be equipped with all the tools and strategies for survival, and to be able to thrive. We want our children to know who they are, deep in the core of their being; to be spiritually, physically, emotionally and mentally aware, to care about their world and other people. This is the identity that matters to us as parents. That our children can own who they are and be proud of who they are. That they can understand how they work and how the world around them works. I often feel we have a double job of preparing our children for the world, while also trying to prepare the world for our children.

At home, within the safety of our family, our children are positively celebrated for their differences; we have a narrative and family identity that makes our differences incredible and admirable. But in school and out in the world, it can be a different matter. Our children often face incredible judgement and bullying.

Family identity is very important. It gives children a sense of belonging – and a sense of belonging and acceptance is a key ingredient for good mental health.

Some identities are birthed in affliction. When we had a child in hospital suffering from suicidal ideation, it led to incredible fear of loss. Every day, cortisol (the body's natural stress hormone) rushed into our new, hypervigilant parent-selves. We desperately checked on our sleeping child morning and night to ensure they were breathing; we felt disconnected from other parents waiting in the school playground. We knew that this experience was changing us, that we would never be the same.

During this time, I became a new type of mother, and David became a new type of father. Then, of course, we had to work out how we were going to work with one another as these newly changed selves. Self-improvement, personal development – these are common phrases these days, and they are seen by some as self-indulgent. For us, they are essential to life. But there is a caveat: for us, self-improvement does not end with self, it extends to where that self fits into the world around us. Self-improvement should raise questions of where we sit within our family and community, and how we live, care for and love our people. It is deeply practical.

DAVID

Identity is complicated. There are so many ways in which we can seek to self-identify: some axiomatic and others felt; some historical and others current. An openness to recognising the changing world around us – and understanding the changing world within us – is essential for our identity to match who we truly are.

The great thing we have discovered about self-identity is that although it begins by resting on historical foundations, it is a pool of potential that our lived experiences are constantly shifting and reshaping. The people we know who are most stuck in the past and express the most indignation about how little resemblance the present bears to their personal 'Golden Age' are those who pointedly – and sometimes proudly – refuse to let their current reality shape their thinking.

When I met Carrie, my life changed in many ways, but perhaps the most profound changes happened because of the way we would talk about who we were. We didn't use the word 'identity', but nonetheless, Carrie was the first person I'd met who was as interested as I was in the 'why'. Not just what I did, but why I did it: why I was the way I was. Her loving acceptance of who I was made me less afraid of showing more and more of the hidden me. We would encourage each other to analyse and challenge the negative stories we told ourselves, or the lies we believed about ourselves and our place in the world. When we first met, like most people, my answer to the question, 'Who are you?' would have been a lot about what I did and actually very little about who I was, where I was from, my values, worldview, failures, hopes, fears, etc. It was not a measurement of me in time and space, in the here and now, but a measurement of what I had done in life. Like many people with low self-esteem, I used my achievements to measure and validate my worth.

The problem is, data has limited value when it comes to identity. I'm a black male. I'm an only child. I'm also one of eight children. I'm a husband, a father, a cousin, a friend. I'm a coach, I'm a mentor, I'm a songwriter, I'm an author, I'm a singer, I'm an MBE. I'm a success or I'm a failure, depending on whose yardstick you are measuring by. All this is accurate, but it's just data, a list of labels; it's not the whole truth, because it tells you very little about my broader identity. Other people may fit this exact profile, yet be totally different to me. Sometimes, people will measure your identity not just by occupation and what you have done in life, but by nationality, gender, or racial or sexual identity – yet this is also not the whole story. Knowing what a person has done in life is only part of the story; the other part is what life has done within that person.

Getting to know each child has done something in me. The idiosyncrasies, needs, gifts and personalities of each child mean that to remain true to my desire to be a good father, I have had to learn and develop. It's an ongoing process. I've had to learn to recognise and respond to the need to be a different father to one child than I am to the others. This is not my natural default; it's been a journey that I couldn't have taken without Carrie's active encouragement.

My upbringing was traditional for a Jamaican home. There was a code of discipline, and consequences for contravening it. There was a predetermined, ideological structure, which my mum gently but firmly tried to impose so that she could bring my life into alignment with her convictions. When Olive was born, I tried to replicate what my mother had done with me. Carrie had also had quite a strict upbringing, so as far as I was concerned, it was going to be straightforward; we were on the same page. Our child was going to be uber-polite, seen and not heard, and a template for any subsequent children we might have. Each would be an impeccably behaved paragon of civility and respect. Before we had children, I knew some cast-iron facts about parenting.

They were all wrong!

What I did find out was that it's so much easier to pontificate on parenting when you don't have children. When no child has rudely declined to fit the pre-set mould you've carefully sculpted for them, it's easy to imagine exactly what they are going to be, and the relationship that will ensue. It was hard to admit that my parenting style needed to change. I couldn't imagine another way of parenting; it was all I knew. I felt somehow that my cultural parenting identity would be compromised if I didn't parent that way. I was so heavily invested in perpetuating a methodology that had worked for me, that I was reluctant to accept that it wasn't working for our children; and when I could no longer deny reality, I was bewildered as to why this traditional method wasn't working. I had to rise above my own cultural scaffolding and meet my children as they were, not as I had imagined they would be. 'Identity parenting' is not a new concept, it's just one with which I was unfamiliar up to this point. A proverb written almost three thousand years ago is a template for identity parenting. It says:

> Start children off on the way they should go,
> and even when they are old, they will not turn from it.[28]

'The way they should go' is individual to each child. It means finding the best in them: their gifts, passions, interests and talents. It means giving them confidence in who they are; it means not incentivising them to become what you want them to be, but discovering who that child really is, their true identity, and then parenting them from that place of reality. It was a world away from my method of imagining what I wanted them to be, and then being disappointed when that idea, which only existed in my expectations, wasn't realised in the real world. Identity parenting required a different way of thinking about each child, and I was reluctant to come to the party. By the time I got there, Carrie was already on the dance floor.

What we are learning along the way

1. Understanding traits is helpful, but tropes are not. Getting an assessment brings clarity.
2. Our sense of identity never stops developing; it's something that we advocate for constantly. And it's also good to know that negative aspects of our identity can be seasonal and can shift.
3. Family or community identity can be wonderful and something to be celebrated.

Questions for the reader to consider

1. How do you see your own identity, and what has shaped your sense of self?
2. How is your current reality shaping your thinking towards yourself and others?
3. Do you share a family or community identity? What does that look like?

3

Identity: Sexuality and Gender

CARRIE

Like David, I'm fascinated by the 'Who are you?' question. I'm intrigued by a person's sense of self and how they came to be who they are.

Human being: the clue's in the title.

To be a human being in a human doing world is a challenge for us all. There is a massive focus on achievement but also behaviour. As adults, we are constantly asked, 'What do you do?' The adult-to-child version of this is 'What have you been up to?' It's all about the verb. The thought of being asked, 'Who are you?' would have most of us recoiling, perhaps because we would find the question too intimate, too intrusive, maybe even a bit creepy, but also because most of us would have no idea how to answer it. If we truly want to understand ourselves, we have to look at what we believe about ourselves. And if we want to see change, then it begins not with behaviour but with who we believe ourselves to be.

People rarely behave out of character. We all behave in ways that tie in with who we think we are, our personal sense of identity. Occasionally, we may notice someone doing something that is out of character for them. We recognise this because we understand who that person is: we understand their behaviours, good and bad, challenging and wonderful, and most of the time they respond to life events as we expect them to. Behaviour is an outworking of identity. Behaviour is communication, the overflow of how someone is experiencing the world around them. If we want to see behavioural changes, there is no point in making a super-long list of rules and regulations. It won't work in the long run. We need to work on *identity* – Who do I believe I am? How do I see myself? – both when we are alone and when we are with others.

Our identities never stop evolving. They are shaped by life events, the choices we make and what we fundamentally believe about ourselves. For our family, there have been some big moments, moments that have made us have to rethink our children and their identities.

Trans Non-binary

One such moment came when Arlo was eleven years old. Back then, they were still known by their birth name. The original name is known as a 'dead name', and people whose names have changed in this way usually hate being called by their dead name. The whole family were sitting in the kitchen after dinner, relaxing, when Arlo stood up as if to make a speech, and announced to the whole family:

'OK, everyone. I just want you to know, I am now a boy, and my name is Ian.'

Before David and I could say anything, the older two shouted a resounding, 'Oh no, not Ian!'

The three of them proceeded to argue the merits and drawbacks of the name, with multiple suggestions for preferred alternatives.

I have to say, I was immensely proud of our family at this moment. There was not a scintilla of judgement, not a beat between the announcement and the response. No shock, no judgement, no negativity. By this point in our parenting journey, David and I had taken on so many changes and differences in our children, we took it in our stride. This was another area about which we would have to learn.

But how should we, as parents, respond to our child telling us they are not the gender they were assigned at birth? Should we take them seriously? Should we tell them they are not allowed to be something other than what we've got them down as? Is this a permanent decision? How quickly do we travel down the road of transition? There are always questions.

How we respond to our children in these immediate, early moments can determine the courses of their lives and their relationships with the family – and, therefore, their identity. Even a hint of disapproval will be read, noticed and taken in. This is why it's so important to think about these things beforehand. What do I think about people being trans? Do I know anything about it? What do I need to know? Plan ahead.

We share a planet with a lot of people who are different from us, and if we want to get along, it helps if we are informed and educated. Personally, we have found it important to think through, enquire and challenge our own thinking. There have been so many surprises with our children, we have come to realise asking ourselves hypothetical questions is important. For us, being prepared meant that in that moment when Arlo spoke up, we were ready with our response.

'Wow, you truly are amazing,' was the gist of it.

The kitchen chat led to them adopting the name Timmy for a while. They then became Mae for a bit, and they are now called Arlo.

I know. It's a lot. We've had to keep up.

One's name is very important, and some may ask, 'Does this make it really hard for them if they keep changing their name?'

Some may say, 'If they're that unsure of their own name they clearly don't know who they are.'

This may be true for them at this age, and it may not, but the most important thing is that they know *whose* they are. They are part of our family, and they are loved and celebrated, and that never changes. That stays the same. We are the constant, the consistent and the solid. If I'm honest, there were at least ten other names that we managed to bat away, so it hasn't at all been a case of 'just going along with it!'

With gender changes, the priority is the child and their thoughts, feelings, beliefs and journey with their identity. At the age of eleven, children can be incredibly fragile, so we wanted to hold the space for Arlo as they processed their thinking. We wanted to make sure we didn't push them down a road if they were simply exploring and discovering; equally, we didn't want to dismiss their ideas about themself and their sense of self. Our job was to walk alongside, and, when appropriate, if appropriate, gently question.

David and I have two big rules for ourselves: firstly, never challenge someone from a place of ignorance, and secondly, we cannot be honest brokers if we have an agenda to change a person's mind. That is not our job. We are there to prompt, to guide, to seek helpful questions that lead to freedom for our children – freedom to be all they are created to be and to sit as comfortably as possible in their own skin. It is possible to celebrate and champion our children and walk positively with them through every step of their development, even while we are working out our own thinking.

We did have questions. Not necessarily for our children, but within ourselves. We wanted to make sure our support of Arlo was right. Studies have shown up to 26 per cent of individuals who present at gender identity clinics have an autism diagnosis;[29] puberty can be traumatic for some young people, and sexual trauma can also play a part. All of this means that one of our jobs as parents is to explore where these feelings of being in the wrong body may come from. These different issues may well cause what is known as diagnostic overshadowing (meaning multiple complex layers), but often it is none of these things, and the person simply knows they are a gender different to the one they were assigned at birth. The space between absolute support and asking those tricky questions has to be navigated gently and held tenderly. It's important to be aware that 92 per cent of trans young people have thought about taking their own lives,[30] so this is not something we can afford to get wrong.

I am aware as we write on this subject that people are highly sensitive to the language used. Using words like 'feelings' (e.g. they feel they are a boy) can be inflammatory and can invalidate a person's 'knowledge' of themselves. For the trans person, it is nothing to do with 'feelings'; it is the absolute belief that this is who and how they have always been. We have had to learn to tread carefully. There has been no handbook for us, and no access to services – although, in our opinions, the Stonewall[31] and Mermaids[32] charities have some very helpful reports and advice on their websites.

There has been no service available to our family, because there is currently a crisis in the NHS regarding meeting the needs of trans young people. With only one – yes, one – gender identity service in the whole of the UK, there were thousands of children and young people waiting for a minimum of two years. In 2020, this one service, operating from the Tavistock and Portman Clinic in London, was found by the Government's Care Quality Commission (CQC) to be inadequate, with inspectors identifying significant concerns.[33] In 2022, that one clinic was closed down. There are plans to create a number of hubs throughout the country,[34] but this is yet to happen – and in the meantime, we, as parents, are pretty much alone in our support of our young people. I do think this needs to be considered when those who support trans children are accused of rushing them towards transition. I have never met anyone for whom a 'rush' has happened.

Often (not always) a trans person will struggle with what's known as gender dysphoria (GD). This is where distress is caused by a discrepancy between a person's gender identity and that person's sex classified at birth (and the associated gender role and/or primary and secondary sex characteristics).[35] The assigned sex is classified at birth based on the appearance of the genitals. The term 'transgender' is used where a person's gender identity is different to their sex assigned at birth. When we were trying to get our heads around this, it initially seemed fairly straightforward: you were a girl, and now you're a boy. However, it's a bit more complicated or nuanced than that. Gender is not binary. Therefore, if your child says they do not believe they are the gender they were assigned at birth, that does not necessarily mean they are now the opposite gender. Some people are gender fluid, with their gender-self being movable and in motion. There are many incremental stages along the continuum of gender, and gender is not just about what you have between your legs.

Studies show that the chromosomes in our bodies are not hard and fast, male and female. Women have two 'X' chromosomes and men have one 'X' and one 'Y'. But science is showing us so much more. According to the journal *Scientific American*, 'New technologies in DNA sequencing and cell biology are revealing that almost everyone is, to varying degrees, a patchwork of genetically distinct cells, some with a sex that might not match that of the rest of their body.'[36] Separate from this, there are also intersex people, those born with the part presence of both sexual systems; for instance, a person may have female genitals outwardly, but have no womb or ovaries and the presence of testes internally. The rates of intersex people have been reported as one or two in 100,[37] but these figures have been contested.[38] There are also a number of studies being undertaken with regards to autism and raised levels of testosterone in those assigned female at birth.

Many people feel very strongly about the gender binary and have issues with trans people. Often, these are people who never interact with trans people but have a need to jump into the fray with an opinion, however unaware they are of the science, or however insensitive to the individual. Some people process with verbal aggression; it's their style. As parents, we want to be aware of every part of the gender argument, but also to be mindful that, for our child, their identity is not up for rabid debate. It's part of their lived reality, not someone else's hypothetical argument.

As it turned out (so far, right now), a few years later, Arlo came out as non-binary. For them, this seems to be a better description of their gender identity.

Missing the Moment

It's 2018, and I am with Olive in our kitchen. I'm cooking; they are doodling in a notebook. They turn the page, write something and turn the book towards me. It's a blank page with the words, 'I am non-binary,' written at the top.

I'm busy, I don't know what it means, and much to my discredit, I say, 'Lovely, darling.'

I ask no further questions. I carry on cooking. I miss the moment. I don't even revisit the subject later. It has so little impact on me that I forget it has even been said. Over the years, I have gone over my reaction many times. What was I thinking? Perhaps I thought Olive was stating they had a new preference or a new view of themselves, and it didn't seem like a big deal; it was like them saying, 'I like cheese.' I had no idea what they were trying to tell me.

A further two years go by, and we are sitting in the garden in 2020. Tylan says, 'Mum, I'm non-binary.'

'OK,' I answer. To be honest, it still means very little to me.

They continue. 'That means my pronouns are now going to be they and them.'

Now they have piqued my interest, because this demands a change from me. I start to look things up online, I do a bit of studying, and I work hard to get the pronoun thing right.

Understandably, Olive is bewildered by my response to their younger sibling, and asks why I'm so keen to get myself educated now when I completely ignored them when they came out.

There are no excuses. Sometimes we get parenting wrong. Sometimes we miss the mark. This was one such occasion. I apologise without reservation.

I had let Olive down. I had shut down the conversation. I had not heard their voice. Thankfully, we have very gracious children.

OLIVE

I remember knowing I was queer my whole life. 'Queer' is an umbrella term used for the spectrum of sexualities and genders. I grappled with my sexuality, but by the time I spoke about it, there wasn't some big 'coming out' moment. It was simply having attraction to people of all genders. At some point, I just happened to tell one person, then two people and three people, then four people, and then kind of everyone knew. But with gender, it was not the same. It was a lot more difficult. It's hard to pinpoint why this was, but, for me, it was probably because the construct of gender is so embedded in our society – to the point that it seems like everything is gendered:

1. colours are gendered
2. words are gendered
3. names are gendered
4. passions are gendered
5. sport is gendered
6. books are gendered
7. jobs are gendered

It's hard to escape the prism of gender.

As a child, my uncle and his husband lived with us for a few years, so I think that queerness in terms of sexuality wasn't as difficult for me.

With gender, I had to deconstruct something in myself in order to come out as non-binary. It wasn't just about my identity; I was grappling with the potential lack of acceptance. Plus, I just didn't have access to representation. Maybe I didn't look hard enough, but I had no sense of belonging or being a part of this group of people. I couldn't see where the group of people were.

Moving away from the concept of two hard-and-fast genders felt like I was falling into nothingness. I knew I was moving away from something that felt entirely wrong to me, but I also felt nervous in stepping away from the societal norms and acceptance around the binary.

One day, I found myself going over and over it in my head. I hadn't even vocalised how I felt. I wasn't sitting there thinking, *Well, I'm non-binary.* I wondered how I could tell somebody else I was feeling these feelings. I was confused and absolutely terrified. But there was one thing I was sure of, and it was that I could not go on not living as the person I was.

I called my best friend, and it took me half an hour to even get to the point, because I was crying so much. I tried to say it quietly, and he jumped in and was totally accepting.

And suddenly it felt easy.

It went from being the hardest thing in the world to suddenly being – OK.

It was OK.

My friend had accepted what I'd just said.

It was still a long time after that until I began to be as open as I am now. There was the incident in the kitchen with my mum where it just didn't land as it should have.

It was during the pandemic where things really began to shift. Before the different pronouns were available on Instagram, I decided to put 'they/them' in my bio. It felt like a huge decision. It shouldn't have, but I thought, *Oh my gosh, I'm coming out to the entire world and everyone's going to judge me,* even though most people probably didn't even notice.

It felt like a big move, because I knew that once I had done it, there was no going back. I couldn't hide again. I thought, *Now people are going to see me for who I am, and they might not accept me.*

I think that's a real fear for some of us. The fear that people will see who I am, and that they will not accept me. It's really terrifying.

I don't know if this is the same for everyone, but for me, maybe because of being black and because of being neurodivergent, I spent a lot of time trying to figure out ways to be accepted and trying to monopolise on the facets of my personality that were the most palatable and acceptable and lovable and fun.

Now, here I was, doing something for myself, where there

was a risk that everyone could think I was nasty, not accept me, or think I was weird or whatever.

It was scary.

It was a turning point for me, because it wasn't just about my gender identity. It was about considering myself and considering being myself before I consider pleasing other people.

Pronouns and Image

CARRIE

It was in 2020 that all three of our daughters became simply children: the she/hers became they/thems, they/hims or he/hims, and we began a new journey of discovery. We were to discover that being non-binary is about so much more than pronouns. It is a view of self, but it also challenges the wider binary nature of our understanding of the world in which we live.

Black and white, the goodies and the baddies, yes or no, binary thinking. Where some people find these absolute opposites helpful and 'holding', like a life scaffolding, there are also many who find them to be incongruent with their life experience. People are rarely all good or all bad. We are complex creatures with grey areas and contradictions. There is actually a great freedom to be found when one lets go of the binary; a beauty arises when we stop judging people as one thing or the other. But black-and-white thinkers can feel threatened by what feels like a total lack of boundaries.

We have learned to embrace the grey. Being non-binary is nothing new. It is not a twenty-first-century construct.

It's simply a contemporary way of describing a section of humanity who have existed since the earliest of times. In Mesopotamian mythology, among the earliest written records of humanity, there are references to types of people who are neither male nor female. Sumerian and Akkadian tablets from the second millennium BCE and 1700 BCE describe how the gods created these people, their roles in society, and words for different kinds of them. In Native American pan-tribal culture, there were more than one hundred different gender expressions and five separate genders were recognised.

Our children have taught us so much; we are truly indebted. I have also worked out that Olive is happy to explain things to me so that I can understand more, Tylan less so, and that's OK. I can read up on things where I have gaps, and allow myself to be corrected when I get things wrong. We have had to learn the meanings of a lot of new words, and a lot of new ideas, too. Cis means 'on the same side as', and in the area of gender, the word 'cisgender' is used (pronounced sis-gender). It's a term that means whatever gender you are now is the same as that you were assigned at birth. Being non-binary is sometimes also referred to as being 'genderqueer' or 'agender'. Being non-binary is not being a third gender in the middle; it is all – or some of – a spectrum. It stands outside the binary.

Some people have asked us if our children are just copying one another or 'doing it to be trendy'. Honestly, no one would choose to have gender dysphoria; no one would choose to be misgendered day after day, often by the same people. No one would willingly choose to be pushed into having to defend their position and their personhood, or to be subjected to the rampant anti-trans tirade promulgated by much of the media. Of all the parts of identity we have encountered, it seems the trans non-binary area really riles people. Cis people will sometimes focus on their own struggle to get pronouns right or the challenges they perceive in having to accommodate trans non-binary people, complaining that they hate having to use 'they' instead of 'she' or 'he' because it's 'bad' English.

When it comes to image, non-binary people dress in every way you can imagine. They do not owe the world androgyny. They may look feminine (fem), masculine (masc) or neutral in the way they dress – and this may vary on different days. It's irrelevant; what's important is who they are on the inside.

The anti-trans voice is loud and intimidating, and is directed at trans non-binary people from a whole host of sources, including from some areas of the radical feminist movement. Women's issues still matter, we women still have such a long way to go in achieving equality, but I do not believe that trans non-binary people threaten or detract from this fight. Each of us may have different life experiences, but it doesn't have to become a competition for who has suffered the most in the fight for equality. If we are compassionate and empathetic towards all people, then the outcomes will favour all people. Hatred towards trans people has no place in the fight for female equality.

Something we have encountered that, to be honest, has shocked us, is people asking about our children's genitals and secondary sex characteristics.

'Will they be having surgery?'

'Will they grow a beard?'

'Will they get rid of their boobs?'

Whether or not our children choose to have top surgery,

take testosterone or have genital reconstruction is no one else's business.

Intersectionality and the Multiple Layers of Identity

Another area people get very confused by is the difference between gender and sexuality. One's sexual preference is different from one's gender identity. In recent years, the word 'queer' has been used to cover a whole range of sexualities and gender identities. Our four children have a range of sexualities.

Whether we are talking race, neurodivergence, sexuality, gender, disability or adoption, defining people by only one part of who they are is problematic. It depersonalises, distils and diminishes them. It puts people into categories, reducing a person to a 'type', meaning we no longer have to consider their essential self. When we look at our children, we do not only see autistic or mixed race, non-binary, trans or gay: we simply see Olive, Tylan, Arlo and Nathan.

Having said this, if we truly desire to understand another person's experience of the world, knowing what they experience and how they interface with the world is helpful. Back in 1989, civil rights advocate and pioneering scholar Kimberley Crenshaw[39] coined the term 'intersectionality' to describe the double oppression black women face in being both black and female, facing both racism and gender discrimination. In 2015, the word entered the *Oxford English Dictionary*.[40] The term is now used more widely to describe those who have two or more areas where they may face oppression.

I think Olive alluded to this in their earlier writing: the more intersections there are, the more we or our children struggle to make ourselves palatable to others. This is not just an issue of people-pleasing or fitting in; it is about wanting to belong. Inside, we are asking, 'Will you allow me to show up as myself?' and 'Am I too much?'

Awkward Situations

There are times when we are attempting to help people to understand our family and we know the person is feeling uncomfortable or simply hasn't been exposed to whatever it is our children are. For example, if the person is white and my autistic child has their hair out in an afro, I can sometimes feel a slight discomfort emanating from the other person (72 per cent of eighteen- to twenty-four-year-olds surveyed have experienced this first-hand in the form of microaggressions when they wear their hair naturally).[41] Perhaps that person is having to make a bit more of a journey to find the shared ground. I may be projecting my own fears or my own attitudes here, but I do experience this from time to time. It's a felt experience, and we talk about it in our family.

When we meet a friend we haven't seen for a while, I often hear, 'Oh, hi. Carrie, your daughter gets more beautiful by the year, doesn't she?'

Sometimes, I notice the over-friendly tone, the person trying to ensure we know they accept us.

I then have to say, 'Actually, they have now changed their name to Tylan, and they are a man.'

It's difficult.

In those moments, something hangs in the atmosphere.

Inside, I am saying, *Please make the journey over. Please say something right now that affirms my son.*

Inside, I am worrying that the person needs time to take in what I have just said and come up with a good response. I can feel Tylan next to me, waiting . . . or, perhaps, observing.

Observing both me and the person. I want Ty to know I am fiercely proud of him, but I don't want to come across as performative or over-trying.

Of course, our old friend is caught off guard. Exposed. This exposure can cause a range of reactions. In a microsecond, they have to readjust their thinking. They may have managed to fix their 'I like black people' face, but they weren't aware there was another shock round the corner. Some people will feel defensive because the exposure is too intense.

'Well, that's wonderful, Tylan. And very handsome you are, too.'

There's a collective sigh of relief.

It is not always like this; sometimes these meetings are comfortable, casual conversations with no underlying narrative. But in conversations like the above, many unspoken words lie behind the spoken. A whole mindset has, perhaps, been challenged. It's as though this person has travelled across a bridge and into our family's world.

We were not hard to reach. We were standing, smiling, with arms outstretched.

Mindset change can take time. For David and me, in our own growth, we know first and foremost that we are committed to filtering our inner questions through love, compassion and truth. Even our hard-wired beliefs have to come under the microscope of love and compassion. There is never any question of us not accepting or affirming our children, but it may take a while for our own inner narratives to catch up with the present. There have been times when David turns his phone towards me, revealing a pop-up photo, an 'on this day in 2012' moment.

And there, before us, is one of our children, pretty as a picture, cute as a button: a little girl confidently smiling to camera. We feel bad for loving the photo, like we have somehow betrayed our child by feeling sentimental. Those days are gone, they are behind us. All that matters is who that child is now.

And somewhere in the back of my mind, I hear a little voice saying, *I'm still here. Look! I grew up and this is who I am. This is who I always was, but there was a journey, remember?*

And I think, *Oh yes, I remember now.* And as I think of my child's gorgeous adult face and the pride I feel at their very being, I am at peace.

Honest Brokers

DAVID

Discovering, understanding and embracing personal identity is one of the most profound, essential and liberating journeys anyone can take. We are all more than a combination of our DNA; we are all more than an amalgam of our influences. We are constantly developing and evolving human becomings. Our core values are often imprinted and set early in life, but the outworking and expression of them changes as we change. If we are the same at forty-five as we were at twenty-five, we've wasted twenty years of potential growth. As our children and young people embark on their journeys, we, as parents, are seldom in a neutral position.

When it came to the subject of sexuality and our parenting journey, it was Arlo, once again, who led the way.

'Mum and Dad, I need to talk to you. This is important. I know you are going to disapprove of what I am about to say. I know you are Christians and God won't agree with me, but I need to tell you: I'm gay.'

We were quick to respond. 'Thank you so much for letting us know, Arlo. This must have been very hard to share, but we are so proud of you. Your sexuality is your business, and we love you and accept you whatever your preference. And, as a matter of fact, we think God feels the same way about you, too.'

Arlo seemed delighted with this response.

They then went to Olive's bedroom to 'break the news'.

From here, they went to Tylan's bedroom and made the same announcement.

Every response was affirming.

We thought that was the end of the 'coming out' announcement, but no.

The next day, Arlo did exactly the same thing again, but more emphatically, particularly with regards to how Carrie and I would disapprove of and condemn them.

Again, we enthusiastically gave them resounding support.

The same thing happened the next night.

They came out every day for a week!

What did this tell us as parents? Somewhere along the line, their learning or experiences had led them to expect condemnation. Even though their gay uncles lived with us for a few years and had their wedding reception in our home, still Arlo expected to be judged negatively. Perhaps school friends had taught them to expect condemnation;

social media stories certainly had. Or perhaps they assumed Carrie and I would have a very conservative Christian view on sexuality. (We don't.)

For us, there wasn't a challenge. In fact, the only challenge was that we'd had a strict 'no boys upstairs in bedrooms' rule. Now we had to extend that to girls . . . and, even more recently, to non-binary guests! The children of this generation are growing up with an outlook on sexuality that is broad and fluid.

What we do or say, just as much as what we don't do or say, serves to either inhibit or liberate our children as they discover who they are. The reality is that many parents choose to bar their children's paths to self-discovery. They may be loving parents who are simply trying to protect their children or guide them along what they see as a safer, more acceptable path. Yet what might be seen to us as 'correct' may not be the right path for our children. This doesn't, in any way, diminish or invalidate the life experience and wisdom that we, as parents, bring to the table. But, like every generation that has gone before, we have much to learn in order to catch up with how our young see the world.

In our family, we have had to learn the many and varied forms of sexuality. Pansexual, asexual, bisexual, queer, straight – all of these terms have different connotations and preferences. We must also remember that they are filtered through how each person conceptualises sexuality, or even differentiates sex and love. Again, this thinking may be different if your child is neurodivergent. If someone's thinking is outside the box, then it follows that their concept of sex, love and gender *may* also be outside the box.

In seeking to walk alongside our children in their growth and development with their sexuality and gender, there is an opportunity to hold the space for discussion. We try to play the role of 'honest brokers': people to whom our children can speak without fear of judgement and condemnation, guiding when guidance is sought, but not insisting. For me and Carrie, there is no pre-set ideal way for our children to be, no gold standard, and no disappointment for us as parents. More than anything, we have learned the value of encouraging our children to be able to show up as themselves.

There comes a point in every parent–child relationship where there is a gradual moving through dependence to interdependence to independence. It's essential to acknowledge that the long-term maintenance of our connection and influence in our child's life is best served by us as parents choosing to go with this process, allowing and even encouraging this gradual transfer of control. The alternative is that our children have to wrestle it from us. It is far healthier that we have a gradual but willing handover to our children, in partnership with them, rather than making them fight us for every inch of ground.

We know that the journey towards a true understanding of self is continual. This means that at key developmental stages, if we embed within a child or young person the idea that who they are at this point is unacceptable, it can greatly damage their self-esteem. In doing so, we are creating a recipe for their future trauma and condemning them to spending years of their adult life trying to mend the fractured pieces of their self-worth. As parents or carers, we have a unique place in the lives of the children in our charge; our words carry weight. Words of rejection and condemnation can penetrate, move in and take up permanent residence in the hearts of even the most resilient children.

Any differences our children might present, whether they be neurological or behavioural, or to do with gender, sexuality, faith, etc., must be filtered through love and acceptance. Without love and acceptance, these differences are seen as anomalies that must be corrected – or, even worse, rejected altogether. Consequently, all too often, children end up feeling invalidated and estranged. Filtered through love and acceptance, differences are simply that: differences, no more, no less. They are indicators of our children's individual identities, not errors to be 'fixed' or problems to be solved.

As parents and carers, so much of our headspace is given over to our hopes, dreams and aspirations for our children's future. Because we have already walked the life miles they are currently navigating, we can see the potential hazards that may lie ahead for them – and yet, as hard as we may try, we can't protect them from life. We can only prepare them for it. A big part of this preparation lies in us acknowledging and accepting our children for who they are, even if it's different from who we wanted or expected them to be. We have all grown in the process.

What we are learning along the way

1. To listen more.
2. To get ourselves educated.
3. To walk alongside our children's evolution.

Questions for the reader to consider

1. How will you respond – or have you responded – to the area of gender and sexuality?
2. Are you aware of where your child is with regards to this subject?
3. Have you created – or can you create – an atmosphere where they can talk to you about this subject?

4

Identity: Race and Culture

DAVID

I was born in Kingston – not the smart London suburb, but the capital of Jamaica. I was born to a single mother who lived with her mother, my gran, although much of my early life was spent in my great-grandmother's two-roomed breeze-block home in the countryside, surrounded by fields, north of the capital. Three generations of women and a little boy; I was the centre of everybody's world. I don't remember much about my great-grandmother, but I do remember she had very long, very shiny, straight, black hair. She was elderly and, as a result of two strokes, spent most of her day in bed, where I would sit chatting with her for hours. I led a happy if somewhat solitary life in the house, but the fields beyond were my playground and held a whole world of discovery.

My earliest memories are of the incredible emotional environment these women created. I can remember feeling safe and loved and quite content being alone, knowing I was held in mind by generations of family. When we were all together, I loved to listen to their conversations. And boy, could they chat – about anything, with gargantuan passion. They were razor sharp and had an innate ability to jump from story to story but somehow still manage to keep up with one another. As a result, I quickly developed a vast vocabulary. I also learned to argue a point. Even as a toddler, I could argue the case for sweet potato over yam like an Old Bailey KC, as if life depended on it. For better or worse, it's a skill I have not lost. Alongside these assets, my ancestors gifted me an inheritance of uproarious laughter and the empathy of a seasoned psychotherapist.

My gran was the first to move to the UK. People didn't just fly in and out back then. When they set sail on the *Empire Windrush*, they were at sea for a month. They had answered the call of the Motherland, and, like my Jamaican uncles who had fought in the war, they came to serve Queen and country. When Gran set sail, my little unit changed. This is my first real memory of separation. The middle part of my sacred female trinity was missing. Soon after, when I was three, my mum and I boarded a boat to England. I was never to see my great-grandmother again; there came my first memory of loss.

Arriving in Southampton in my little summer suit (what other kind would you need in Jamaica?) the first words I uttered on English soil were, 'Mummy, it's cold, can we go home now please?'

In his book *Way of the Peaceful Warrior*, Dan Millman says,

'The secret of change is to focus all of your energy not on fighting the old but on building the new.'[42]

These are wise words articulating an outlook that would serve me well in later life. But the three-year-old boy shivering on a freezing Southampton dock on a wet and windy January morning dressed in summer clothes didn't care about building anything.

In that moment, I expressed a sentiment that would typify my outlook for years to come: *I don't want this new world; I want the old world back.*

As we stood, holding each other to stay warm, my mum knew there was no going back. My great-aunt was the first in the family to emigrate to England. Unbeknown to my mum, she had been saving for years to buy us two one-way tickets. She had taken it for granted that Mum would be delighted, but she wasn't. Mum had had no intention or desire to leave Jamaica, but her auntie had scrimped and saved, gone without, and spent hundreds of pounds on tickets. Auntie would not have been refunded the money, and such was the hierarchical nature of Jamaican family life in the late 1950s that it would have been unthinkable for my mother to refuse. So here we were.

Over the next couple of years, we moved between various parts of east London. The people living around us were almost all in the same socio-economic boat, living from one week's wages to the next, and all working class. In the 1960s, being East End working class put us low down on the food chain, and being immigrants put us even lower. Caribbean immigrants came from different social classes, with differing levels of education and different qualifications. We were not a homogeneous mass, all the same. We came from different islands within the Caribbean and arrived with differing expectations and aspirations, but whether we were university lecturers, manual workers or at any point of the compass in between, stereotypes die hard. To many (but not all) of the white people we encountered, we were just blacks, niggers, wogs and coons; we were considered loud and dirty, unwelcome and unwanted.

Our first home was a rented room in a house in Mile End, owned by a Jamaican couple. My mum would leave for work as a telephonist at the American Embassy at 8am, returning at 6pm. The landlords said I could spend the day with them. We had no TV or radio. At the age of three, the landlords would leave me in our rented room, sleeping or looking at picture books all day, apart from twenty minutes in the middle of the day when I would come downstairs and eat lunch with them. As the winter evenings closed in, I would spend hours staring out of the window, crying, longing for my mum to return. Every day I feared that perhaps she never would. I had gone from being part of a very close, attached family to being completely alone and feeling abandoned.

Mum, aware that I wasn't being well looked after, mentioned our predicament to friends at church, hoping, perhaps, for comfort and support – but she got much, much more. A white English couple, the Bomfords, offered to take me in from Sunday night to Friday night. Marge and George had a house in Forest Gate. They had two sons, who were three years and one year older than me. George, the dad, worked in an office, and his wife was a seamstress working from home. I was with the family for a year. While the sons were out at school, I spent many happy hours sitting beneath Auntie

Marge's sewing table, listening to the music on the radio, singing and jabbering about nothing and anything.

With this change, I was fully exposed to a typical white British family, unfiltered and unselfconscious. I discovered, by proxy, what it was like to have siblings, the squabbling and unconscious positioning integral to family life. After a while, I started school. I remember my first months as the only black child; the teachers turned a blind eye to racist playground taunts and bullying, and the Bomford boys acted as my minders. The Bomfords took me in, they made me feel safe, and for five nights a week, for a whole year, I became part of them: part of what, in the 1960s, was recognised as a 'proper' family. I was introduced to the concept of there being different types of family and different understandings of what family meant. To the Bomfords, it was Mum, Dad and two kids; to me, it was just me and my mum. But that was about to change again, when we moved in with my gran. I left the safety, warmth and comfort of the Bomfords' home and returned to being part of an intergenerational family.

Gran lived in Dalston, on the attic floor of a large, damp, mice-infested Victorian house. When Mum and I moved in, we brought the total to seventeen occupants, sharing one bathroom with no hot running water. But at least the toilet was inside. Gran, Mum and I occupied one fair-sized room, which we partitioned off to separate the living area from the sleeping area. The landing, which had an ancient four-ring hob and oven, served as the cooking area. There were two cupboards on the landing, one with a butler sink, where we washed up the dishes, and another that was a store cupboard, where brooms, mops and tins of food were kept. Across the hall was another room, identical in size and layout, which was shared by Frank Cooper and Samuel Rawlins (Uncle Frank and Uncle Sammy), two young West Indian men who were here to study and work.

Apart from these two, every other room was occupied by a family comprising mother, father and varying numbers of children. Like every West Indian child of my generation, I didn't dare call grown-ups by their first name. They were Mr, Mrs, Miss, Auntie or Uncle. All of us West Indians wanted to make the most of every opportunity we were given. We were creative and industrious. Uncle Frank eventually got married, left for America, and went into business. Uncle Sammy went to Canada, then back to the Caribbean. He got married, stayed in academia and was awarded a Nobel Peace Prize in 2007. But back in the sixties, award or no award, all of us were, at best, just 'coloureds' (the polite nomenclature), with no real power, no status – and, in my case, no father.

A lot of our identity comes through our understanding of where we come from, our family origins and life events. As a child, I knew I was an outsider. It was impossible not to know. On our very first English holiday, to Cliftonville in Kent, when I was seven, Mum, Gran and I arrived at our boarding house to be told we couldn't stay. Our booking had been made by phone, and the landlady hadn't realised we were 'coloureds'. We were told the other guests would leave if they allowed us in. So we carried our suitcases from one boarding house to another, until finally we found one that would take us. We were outsiders, moving through familiar landscapes but never belonging. Our passports said 'British', but the 'ish' was doing all the heavy lifting. That sense of being on the outside looking in became a defining part of my identity. For Mum and Gran, the rejection cut deep; the

Britain they had imagined was so different to the one they encountered.

Each year, 24 May was a big day for West Indians of my mum and gran's generations. It was Empire Day. All over the Caribbean, school children assembled in playgrounds and sang 'God Save the King' (and later, Queen) beneath the Union Jack. It was an annual opportunity to celebrate the monarch, the empire and their part in it. Empire Day was just one of many reminders that they were British, belonging to an empire upon which the sun never set. In Jamaica, the flag was British, their passports were British, and they were ultimately governed from London. They were not citizens, they were subjects, a part of something bigger than themselves, bigger than Jamaica; they were part of the British world. This in turn, engendered in them a sense of belonging to the Mother Country, and they were taught to have a strong sense of pride in their Britishness.

Around half of all soldiers fighting for Britain in the Second World War were from the empire outside the UK: India, Australia, Canada, the West Indies, New Zealand and the African continent. My great-uncles were among those who made their contribution against fascism for the Mother Country. So, when Britain advertised in the Caribbean for workers to help rebuild the motherland after the Second World War, many felt it was their duty to answer the call. With a naive sense of belonging, they left their homes, believing they were going to another home, a place of equal belonging. It didn't take long for their illusions to be shattered. Their labour may have been needed, but their presence was unwanted.

Throughout my childhood, I would encounter people who took it upon themselves to make sure I knew that I wasn't wanted, that this was not my home. The conversations were mind-numbingly predictable.

'Where are you from?'

'Dalston.'

'No, where are you *really* from?'

'Do they live in trees where you're from?'

'Do they throw spears where you're from?'

Or: 'You blacks always smell; you don't wash, do you?' This, among white people, was a widely accepted, seldom-challenged 'fact'. Usually stated by somebody who ate their chips from yesterday's newspaper, as though there was nothing more hygienic than chips with salt, vinegar and two-day-old newsprint ink.

It went on and on, with facts never being allowed to get in the way of a volley of abuse. Eventually, we learned the importance of secrecy, of not giving oxygen to the flames of insult, bigotry and hostility. Most white people already thought themselves superior to us; this meant that if there was anything in our circumstances that they could use against us, they would and did, so we learned to keep things to ourselves. If we went without, nobody outside the family or the community needed to know. If somebody didn't have work, nobody needed to know.

Today the African-Caribbean community is often classified as 'hard to reach'. We aren't hard to reach; we're here, ready and waiting. We just learned from experience that the more people know about you, the more some can and do use it against you. When I met Carrie, her experiences had given her the need for disclosure, because in her upbringing, secrecy had led to a lack of protection. In my upbringing, secrecy was my strongest protection.

CARRIE

I am a white woman married to a black man. I was brought up racist; I can't remember anyone who wasn't racist when I grew up, back in the sixties and seventies. I grew up in north London – Enfield, to be exact. It was suburbia with an identity crisis: too far out of London to be edgy in an 'I know the Krays' kind of way, and not quite close enough to the fields of the shires to be part of the 'we keep horses' set. It was suburbia, the land of twitching net curtains and keeping up with the Joneses. Everything and everyone was either better than or less than; we knew our inferior position in one direction, but we always had someone to look down on in the other.

Meeting David was the defining moment of my life; there is no doubt about that. I was not someone who gave my heart easily. The experiences of my early childhood had taught me to do the very opposite to my mum, who'd had disastrous relationships after my dad left when I was seven. I wanted to have agency, to be strong, to make a life for myself, and for love to happen with a good and stable person who would treat me the way I deserved to be treated. I had two long relationships before David, one lasting five years and one lasting two and a half, and both partners were good, lovely guys who have gone on to have strong marriages.

My mum remarried when I was thirteen. She met my stepdad on a blind date, and they were head over heels in love, real soulmates. This was a great, close-quarters example of marriage for me. My stepdad truly adored my mum, and I knew this was the kind of healthy relationship I wanted. But we'd never talked about the colour of my future husband. I was simply expected to marry a white guy.

To me, the concept of love at first sight is utterly ridiculous, and yet there was something of this in meeting David. When our eyes met for the first time, it was as if I had come home. *Oh, hello, I know you*, went through my head. It was the weirdest experience, as if we had looked straight into one another's souls, holding the very present moment right alongside destiny. There was no emotional attachment to this experience, no deep love, not even a sense of sexual attraction at that point; it was more than that. It was a knowing in my deepest self. I gave David my phone number, but fear got the better of him and he didn't call for a couple of weeks. I was surprised, but I wasn't sitting by the phone, waiting. I wasn't remotely disappointed; I was just a bit confused. A little voice in my head said, *Years from now, you'll be married with children, and you'll look back and think, this is the man you should have married.* Now, where that thought came from, I have no idea, but there was something very special from the start with us. When he did eventually call me, we picked up where we had left off. It was as though we had known each other for years.

David is like no other person I have ever met. He is creative, funny, intelligent, spiritual and romantic. When we got together, it was a unique experience for me. He brought out a playful side in me; he challenged me intellectually, emotionally and spiritually, and introduced me to a whole new culture.

My first family meeting was with David's gran, a beautiful, white-haired lady with wisdom to match her years – all seventy-eight of them. David's mum was living back in Jamaica by then, so the initial family approval would come from his grandmother. Gran was a force. She was hilarious, a great listener, an unashamedly forthright speaker and a real character. She was absolutely loved, and the family had to share her with the whole of Tottenham – she was 'Gran' to everyone who knew her.

I had never been into a West Indian home, and my early memories are of huge quantities of mouth-watering food – plantain, yam, sweet potato, rice and peas, fried chicken – all followed by washing-up, sharing, laughter and deep conversation. There were plastic covers on the arms of the sofas and crocheted doilies over the backs; there were cabinets full of trinkets and photos of every relative who had ever lived. This was also my first experience of a concept David and I would go on to adopt, the *open house*. There was always a pot on the stove with something delicious to eat, and always enough food for anyone who showed up. Gran would invariably send me away at the end of the day with some treat or gift which she would put inside a bag, within a bag, within another bag . . . it was like pass the parcel.

Gran had a strong Jamaican accent, and I would concentrate hard, following the stories of her life. She was mesmerising. She had the ability to make you feel as though you were the only person in the room; she always had time for you and was interested in what you had to say. This is something I think David inherited when it came to our relationship. Gran would pass away just five years later, and I still treasure the fact that I had those years to get to know her. I also met the rest of the family, who were a total treat. David's family have had such an influence on me and have shaped so much of my life.

But what did I feel in my heart in those early days? In this fully exposed and privileged place of truly encountering a black extended family? All my childhood teaching was up in the air. I felt a deep sense of shame about my racist thinking. I don't mean I had to deal with hatred or anything that strong, but I had grown up with a sense of superiority, with what today we would call white privilege. I had overlooked this incredible community. When I think about my attitude before meeting David, it honestly makes me cry. I could not have met a nicer, more welcoming family. They invited me into their home and accepted me. They fearlessly showed me love, and to this day, I am still utterly humbled by the experience. British West Indians are a unique community, with incredible experiences and history. For me, they define so much of what it means to belong. My West Indian family and friends created an epic-scale mindset change in me.

On my side of the relationship, I would have to expose David to the judgement of my parents. Breakfast in our family home was tea, toast and the *Daily Mail.* My parents had 'gone up in the world', living in Hertfordshire; my stepdad was men's captain of the golf club, and my mum was ladies' captain of the tennis club. My parents were never going to be rude to David; they were never going to shout racist abuse or cause a scene. Their response was a type of insidious racism that crept its way into conversation in subtle ways. They, too, had a lot to confront and a lot of changing to do.

It's hard not to like David. He is charming and interested and confident yet humble. He walked into my family home and threw his arms around my stepdad, much to my stepdad's surprise, and something I hadn't managed to do in the seven years since he'd married my mum. David also hugged my mum and respectfully called her Mrs Gabriel, until she gave permission to use her first name. Much as they were trying not to, my parents liked him. I could see this was causing an existential crisis in them!

For the next two and a half years, until David and I got married, my parents would try to introduce conversations where they could let me know how they felt without being explicit: 'What do you think about having children? I'm not sure about mixed-race children. Do you think it's fair on them?' was a regular one.

Just as I had, but on a much bigger scale, they were trying to process their own thinking. Then things got a whole lot more serious.

Two months before we were due to marry, my mum stood in my bedroom doorway and said, 'You cannot marry him. I won't give my approval, and I don't want him in the house.'

This was a crucial test for me and one that I was determined not to repeat when I had my own children. A lot of my formative years were spent as the child of a single parent, so my mum's approval of me mattered more than anything in the world. If I was going to be with David, I would have to make a choice. I would have to cut the emotionally controlling umbilical cord between me and my mother, whatever the cost. I gently called her out on her racism and very calmly made it clear that I was marrying David, and that was that. For the next three days, the atmosphere in our family home was dreadful. No one spoke. If I entered a room, my parents would find some reason to leave it. I was being given the silent treatment. On day three, David came to pick me up in the car. I got in the passenger side, but before we could drive away, my mum rushed from the house and pulled the driver's door open. I had no idea what was about to happen, and I was afraid.

I need not have been. My mum threw her arms around David, almost pulling him out of the car. 'I'm so, so sorry. Please forgive me. I cannot believe how I have treated you, and this is not how I feel. I love you. Please come into the house.'

I am still pained and inspired by David's response. He was gracious to her undeserving soul. He would pay the price for her growth by being generous-spirited in the face of hatred. These days, I am horrified to see our black community still having to do this in countless ways. I really question why they have to do all the work. The weight of a generous response should not be for our black community to carry. The heavy lifting and onus of responsibility belongs with us as white people; we are the ones who need to make changes, consistently and without compromise.

As we talked things through with my parents, it transpired that members of my mum's tennis club had been telling her it was disgusting that I was with a black man. They had questioned her, asking her why wasn't she doing anything about it? Why hadn't she thrown me out of the house? My parents, who had always wanted to escape the city and fit in to country life, were facing wrath and judgement from their own community. From that day, my mum and stepdad became our fiercest defenders and allies, standing up to comments and calling out racism.

David's mum also had a lot of reservations about me. David had been married before, and she didn't trust his judgement. She found it hard not to step in, to advise and criticise, so David had his own journey to make, and his own emotional umbilical cord to cut by standing up to parental control. Thankfully, by the time we got married, all parties were on board, and both mums became new mums for each partner. I adored David's mum; she was a real inspiration to me. She was insightful, supportive and wise, and became a total cheerleader for our relationship.

The day we married was the best day of my life. I felt like I was the first person to ever discover love, and I wanted to shout it from the rooftops. We had cracked the code; dreams come true; real, romantic love exists. With no consistent template for marriage, we could make it up. We could become everything we needed to be for ourselves and each other. David and I were madly in love. There have been so many times I have tried to work out how this happened. Neither of us had any part to play in how we found one another or why it works for us. I just know I still want to spend every day of my life enjoying what he brings and trying to make his life better. That feeling has never gone away. In fact, it has increased over the years.

Our early love grew roots downwards, and branches upwards and outwards, creating vast networks of interests and people, building whole communities. Our 'open house' outlook created a village. And into that village came our children.

DAVID

So, you'd like to think things have changed with regards to race; after all, it's been over three decades since Carrie and I got married. During lockdown, we saw that huge divisions still exist in our world – and we saw just how deep they are. The death of George Floyd caused a worldwide spectrum of response. One of the things we heard over and over was:

'It's different in the UK; we are not like America.' To an extent, that's true – but only to an extent. The overt 'Go back to where you came from' kind of racism of the sixties and seventies became largely consigned to the fringes during the nineties. I wish I could say racism had been eradicated altogether, but for many, it was just hiding in the shadows, waiting to be legitimised. Political events in Europe, America and Britain have seen phrases and attitudes many of us dared to hope had been relegated to the dustbin of history re-enter the common discourse. We discovered racism wasn't just the comfort blanket of a small and diminishing minority; it wasn't dying as some of us had been led to believe in the 1990s and 2000s. No, it was just hibernating beneath a thin veneer of civility, and once that sheen was rubbed off, once that prejudice was re-legitimised, what lay beneath was just as ugly as it had ever been.

Whether from government, institutions or members of the public, our community faced racism. From 2014, immigration law changed, and the Windrush scandal happened. Members of my community who had lived here for decades were put on airplanes and 'sent home'. How did something like this happen? Many of our Windrush generation had lost documentation, or as children, had simply never had any. The story of Renford McIntyre demonstrates one such atrocious example of the treatment of our West Indian community.[43] Renford worked and paid taxes here for forty-eight years. He was an NHS driver and a delivery man, but in 2014, he was asked for his updated paperwork from his employers. This revealed that he did not have documents showing he had a right to be in the UK. As a result, he lost his job. Having no job meant he was forced to seek housing and social assistance.

Unfortunately, he faced the same problem with this, and eventually ended up homeless. He put together four decades' worth of documents, including HMRC, national insurance and NHS pension records. He sent these to the Home Office, but they were not satisfied. This was following the 2012 interview in which the then-Home Secretary Theresa May talked to the *Telegraph* about directing the Home Office to create a hostile environment.[44]

And hostile it was.

It's difficult to measure the impact of this on the Caribbean community. We were in shock. Yet again, we felt unsafe. The aftermath of the Brexit referendum has seen an increase in antagonism towards immigrants and non-white Brits, and a growing attitude of hatred towards asylum seekers. The impact of this has been felt by many people of colour living in the UK.

Racism spreads and infests, and before we know it, individuals become confident enough to speak out about their views towards non-white individuals. I found this out first-hand when I had two obvious encounters with racism recently.

To give the stories some context, when walking our dogs, I try to stay within ten minutes of home, so that if anything kicks off, as has happened on numerous occasions, Carrie knows I'm close. This means that to make up the distance the dogs need to walk, I take them into and out of nearby cul-de-sacs and blocks of flats, as well as along the main roads. Just after lockdown ended, I encountered a problem. It was late at night, and a middle-aged man in a Volkswagen tailed me very slowly for a couple of minutes as I walked along the road. If that wasn't sinister enough, he then pulled up a little ahead of me, lowered his window and began shouting racist abuse at me, accusing me of walking my dogs down his road so that I could look inside people's cars before coming back to steal them. He then said if he saw me walking down his road again, he'd beat me up. He opened his car door as if to get out, before his passenger implored him not to, at which point he drove off.

I was shaken and confused, as I didn't know what he was talking about. But most of all, I was angry. Angry that he had hurled racist abuse at me. Angry that instead of seeing a middle-aged man walking his dogs, like so many others I'd seen on the same route, he saw a black man. He had made it clear that he'd arrived at his conclusion based on the colour of my skin. I was angry because it took me right back to east London in the 1970s, to an era and an attitude I thought I'd left behind. But hey, it was one crazy person, right? Just one incident. Or so I thought, until a few weeks later.

I was walking the dogs along a completely different road, less than five minutes' walk from my house. Three older white men were huddled together having a chat. As I passed them, the largest one said, 'What are you doing, walking down here?' Politely, I answered that I was walking my dogs, that I'd been on that road many times before, and that it was a public road. 'Well, we don't want your kind down here, now f*** off!'

There's an old Jamaican saying: 'It's better to humour a fool than to vex him.' Taking that advice to heart, I turned and walked away, exiting to the soundtrack of choice racist insults from the big man and his friends.

There's a postscript to this last event. A few weeks later, I was walking along the same road, and I saw the same man, this time on his own.

'Excuse me,' he said.

I stopped, not knowing what to expect.

'Sorry about the other day, I didn't recognise you. One of the blokes you saw me with is a bit racist, I was actually making things better for you, he'd have made matters much worse.'

He then went on to tell me how much his wife liked mine; that she worked with neurodiverse children and had been horrified at the way they had treated me. And although I felt safer, knowing he wasn't going to attack me, his words didn't make me feel any better. They were a throwback, a reminder of when children at school would say, 'I don't like blacks, but you're OK.'

Making exceptions because this one is your friend or that one is on the telly doesn't make someone less racist. It just makes the person selectively racist.

I know, having told this story, that there will still be people who will say, 'But that's just individuals, not the system or the institutions.' As a dad, I want to gather my children and hold them close, to keep them safe and protected from these kinds of experiences. I am disempowered, knowing that I can do very little except perhaps prepare and help them in their understanding. And in response to this, here's a reflection Olive wrote a week after George Floyd's death in 2020, during lockdown.

OLIVE

There is a certain numbness that is required of black people, to keep going, to find joy, freedom and expansion within a world that often appears to want to crush us.

In the wake of George Floyd's murder, many systems were

called into question. Seeing the systems that I have suffered under being exposed and called out daily on national TV impacted me. It removed the thick lid I had placed carefully over racial trauma and pulled those feelings rapidly to the surface.

When I was first verbally racially attacked in primary school, I think I believed that when I got older things would get better. Maybe being raised in a house where blackness and black culture was celebrated and invested in led me to believe that the world I was growing into might be the same. Maybe it was just school or the parents of the kids in my school, and maybe once I entered an artistic environment full time things would get better.

I don't consider myself particularly optimistic per se, but when disappointment happens in this area it hits like a punch, and I'm thrown; my inner voices yelling at me to lower my expectations. The racialised abuse at drama school – and at times the entertainment industry writ large – came as a hard disappointment.

There is still deep unlearning and a radical shift needed for change to come. I believe this change cannot happen without black people's voices being front and centre of that conversation.

CARRIE

I honestly believe there is a desire among many people to find a place of inclusion, but the way in which this happens will demand awkward conversations and a robustness on the part of the person or system needing to make the changes.

For example, in an area such as film and TV we have seen

a massive shift towards the inclusion of black and mixed-race actors, but there is still a long way to go. If you take the simple and innocuous subject of the hair and make-up departments, more often than not, you will find black actors being made up by an artist with no training on how to make up any skin tone other than white – and most don't have even a basic idea of how to work with afro hair. You can find a cast with multiple black and mixed-race actors but with not one black or mixed-race make-up artist who would understand their needs. A black or mixed-race make-up artist will know how to make up every skin tone, yet a white make-up artist will most likely not have had the training to work with any skin tone or hair styling other than that of white artists.

I have spent years watching David being patted down with 'white skin tone' powder. I have watched my children on many sets being patted down with powder for someone several shades darker. I have witnessed their afro hair being mismanaged, with no afro hair products in the department or with products being used incorrectly, and professional hair and make-up artists with no idea how to style afro hair even in the most basic way. I have seen make-up departments where the answer to the lack of training is simply to make their black and mixed-race female actors wear wigs. I have heard many comments while the actor is sitting in the chair on 'how hard their hair is', 'how difficult it is to style', or questioning why they need so many hair products. Often, black and mixed-race actors are expected to turn up for work with their hair already done or to do their hair themselves, using their own products.

In any profession or situation, an environment needs to be created where black and mixed-race people can ask for changes without being seen as a bother, demanding, aggressive or ungrateful. In fact, ideally, we need colleagues and teams to understand their needs, without the person having to worry about this stuff. The constant need to explain and educate can be exhausting.

A level of empathy is required by those who hire and those who have decision-making roles. If they can be ahead of the game this helps. Why wait for members of any of our marginalised communities to have to pluck up the courage to speak up? Why not use one's imagination to think about how the people around us may be experiencing the world, the environment and the situations they find themselves in?

DAVID

The death of George Floyd and the emergence of the Black Lives Matter movement divided opinion. On the one hand, many black people were accused of ingratitude and a lack of proportion. After all, we are told, 'Things like this don't happen in the UK,' and 'Don't *all* lives matter?' I've lost count of how many times I switched on the TV to see a group of white people debating the black experience. There were people who, during this time, made themselves known to be allies, people who were horrified to hear about the treatment of the black community and who stood up to the racists. These people are so helpful for our community; we need allies.

In Britain, black people are in the minority. When any minority is disadvantaged, it is quite possible for the majority to be blind to their suffering and deaf to their cries. By taking a minority issue, like structural racism, out of the margins and putting it up front and centre, it became impossible to ignore. The killing of George Floyd and the footage of his murder was seen all over the world; it provided a focal point and the catalyst for a global, multi-ethnic, anti-racist movement represented by the words 'Black Lives Matter'.

Inevitably, there were white people who felt awkward, threatened and defensive. In our society, anyone who is biracial is categorised as black, making Carrie the only white person in our family. Carrie has witnessed first-hand the myriad subtle ways that people of colour can experience different treatment. Being working class and having lived through times when money was tight, Carrie recognised that 'white privilege' doesn't mean that white people haven't worked hard for what they've got or haven't suffered. It means that whiteness comes with an array of benefits not shared by people of colour. White privilege isn't about whether white people are financially or socially disadvantaged – it's unquestionably true that many are. White privilege is about whether people are socially disadvantaged because of their race.

Ironically, the phrase 'white privilege' was coined by a white person, Peggy McIntosh, an American feminist, anti-racism activist, scholar and speaker. In her 1988 essay 'White Privilege and Unpacking the Invisible Knapsack',[45] McIntosh listed forty-six of her own everyday advantages, such as:

- I can go shopping most of the time, pretty well assured that I will not be followed or harassed.
- I can be sure that my children will be given curricular materials that testify to the existence of their race.
- If a traffic cop pulls me over or if the IRS audits my

> tax return, I can be sure I haven't been singled out because of my race.

Through an extensive list of everyday experiences, McIntosh illustrates that white privilege is like an intangible gift of unearned entitlements and advantages – and not just unearned but, by and large, unnoticed.

When you are accustomed to privilege, equality can feel like oppression. When it becomes clear to defenders of the status quo that they are losing ground socially, politically and intellectually, typically they try to reframe the argument. It's long been the tactic of gaslighters to take clearly understood definitions of words or phrases – in this case, 'Black Lives Matter' and 'woke' – and redefine them in a way that makes the phrases seem inflammatory, and opposition to them seem perfectly reasonable. Reframing the argument on their terms made it possible for them to present any issue as a matter of differing opinions, ignoring the mountain of proven evidence that black people are disadvantaged by the colour of their skin. Instead, they made the argument about contentious views, like defunding the police or 'critical race theory'.

There are some who shut down every conversation by accusing others of being 'woke'.

When you look up the word 'woke' in the *Oxford English Dictionary*, it says: 'Woke; adjective: Originally: well informed, up to date. Now the definition has been expanded to include: 'alert to racial or social discrimination and injustice'.[46] The word 'woke' has been in use since the 1960s; it's nothing new. So how have being 'up to date', 'well informed' and 'alert to racial and social injustice' become negative traits? Does this mean being 'anti-woke' makes you ill-informed, out of date and unaware of racial or social discrimination and injustice? There isn't a rule that demands we care about anybody but ourselves; there is no statute that punishes us for not loving our neighbour. In fact, whole political philosophies have been built on the preservation of self-interest, even if it's at the cost of the suffering of others. If they wish, people are entitled to wear their resistance to racial and social equality as a badge of honour.

Woke? To be honest, I'm glad to have been awakened.

The opposite of racist isn't 'not racist', it's 'anti-racist'. What does it mean to be anti-racist? It is the difference between being passive and active. It's the difference between not doing or saying racist things, and actively standing and speaking up against those who do. It's the difference between not laughing at a racist comment, and actually challenging the person making the comment. It's the difference between being neutral and taking a stance. Mere non-racism is the reason the phrase 'silence is violence' exists, because silence, even if we disagree internally, is too easily taken as complicity.

To be anti-racist takes courage, particularly in these times when the accusation of racism is considered to be more offensive than the actual racist act itself. Being anti-racist is a journey that begins with the embracing of the principle that all of us are equal. This, in itself, is not the end goal; it's the starting point. From here, we begin to recognise and challenge racism wherever it's evident, even in ourselves. Once our eyes are opened to this recognition, we will more easily begin to identify the structures and customs that benefit one race of people to the disadvantage of others. If something is wrong and we fail to challenge it, it's vital to remember that whatever we are not changing, we are choosing.

It is also important to ask ourselves what an anti-racist society could look like, and what our part in building it could be. Raising children to be racially inclusive requires not being afraid to talk about race with them. There is sometimes a fear that highlighting race means running the risk of making a big deal out of something children would otherwise be unaware of. However, very young children (even babies) are able to identify differences in skin colour and facial features. By avoiding or shutting down any questions they may have about race, we are creating a taboo around the subject. If a child asks about the colour of someone's skin, it's better to explain that skin colour depends on the amount of melanin someone has in their body. The more they have, the darker their skin; the less they have, the lighter their skin. To a child, this helps to begin making the subject of race one of biology rather than comparative values and social standing. Answering the questions helps to normalise the topic of race.

Race has long been used to justify bias and afford unfair privilege to some while denying equal standing to others. Children are sponges and assume and internalise by osmosis the prejudices that are prevalent in the environment they inhabit. Children often have a real sense of what is fair, and if yours is one such child, support their desire to help make things fair for all, regardless of race. My mother used to say to me, 'We have to speak up when things are not right and when things aren't fair.' It's a message for all children. This is anti-racism in a nutshell. Action, no matter how small, is the foundation on which equity is built.

What we are learning along the way

1. Racism still exists in the UK.
2. To be anti-racist, we have to take positive steps to make change.
3. We still have a long way to go.

Questions for the reader to consider

1. Are you aware of racism you or others may be experiencing?
2. What actions could you take in order to be anti-racist locally?
3. What actions could you take within your family in order to support being anti-racist nationally?

5

Communication and Strategy

CARRIE

Communication is a big part of life, especially as we parent our children.

Trees communicate with each other.

Animals communicate with each other.

Even music and water communicate with one another.

So why is it so darned hard for us humans?

One issue is that when we think of communication, it is often through the tiny form of speech. We have elevated the art of talking to god-like status, and attribute the epithet 'good communicator' to anyone who can fluidly string together sentences, even if those sentences aren't actually communicating anything of substance. In reality, communication is actually happening all around us, and between us, on every level. With the advance of technology, we are receiving information twenty-four hours a day, seven days a week. We have incredible access to one another. Now, with the press of a button, I can translate a text from a friend written in Japanese and know exactly what they wanted to tell me. I can stand in a village in Sierra Leone and call home in London. So, has all this access made us better communicators?

It is interesting to note that the number of people describing themselves as unseen, unheard, overlooked or misjudged seems to be greater in our society now than ever before. Something's clearly not working. Social media has mobilised an army of polemicists, of black-and-white thinkers. Very few are prepared to give time or consideration to perspectives that don't mirror their own, with the prevailing thinking from all sides being, 'We're right, you're wrong; we're good, you're bad.' Like many, our children had an 'Opposites Day' at school – only to discover that this was the world they would inhabit when they grew up. Not only is our thinking polarised, we also bring a tsunami of criticism against those who think differently, heaping shame on the heads of those who have a different opinion or have arrived at different conclusions, and treating all detractors as the enemy.

Sometimes, it feels like the world has forgotten how to communicate.

Watching and learning how our children communicate has been one of the great joys of our lives. They often use words as a last resort. This calls upon David and me to be able to read the room, to feel the space, to discern what is happening without the use of words. It also shapes how we respond, whether we speak or stay silent, communicating in some other form.

When Olive was small, they would walk into our bedroom

in the morning and put their face about an inch from one of ours, then wait. If we stayed silent, they would breathe more heavily, and if we still failed to stir, they would start singing in our faces. Once we were awake, they would jump between us, screaming, 'I'm in the middle!'

I have to be honest; it was the very best way to be woken up. Olive was like a ray of sunshine bursting into our lives. Tylan was more reticent, holding back on the kind of big, cuddly affection we were used to giving. Tylan would sidle into the bed beside me and lie facing outwards. After a while, I began to pop my hand on the pillow next to him and say, 'Tylan, Mr Hand is very tired. Please don't wake him up.'

Then I would feign sleep, while sneakily watching Ty lavish love on my hand, stroking his face with my hand and chatting away ten to the dozen. Every now and again, 'Mr Hand' would face-plant Ty, and he would squeal with delight, backing into me and allowing me to hold him.

Arlo, meanwhile, loves squeezing things, and David's face is Arlo's squeeze toy. They now have long, complicated routines around this form of affection and the bonds are strong.

These moments were the foundation of trust and communication, and a commitment to discovering each child's identity.

Communicating with a child who has had broken attachment demands an even greater level of skill and huge amounts of patience. With adopted children, the movement towards the centre has largely to be dictated by the child. If a child has been neglected or abused, they need to find their autonomy. Every 'ask' we give that child may lead to them feeling criticised, shamed or even abandoned. All communication has the potential threat of calamity.

Our Nathan came to us at the age of two. It was very difficult for him to attach and bond to us, and to trust the attachments. I knew that Nathan was grieving the loss of his foster-carer, whom he had been with from the age of about four months to two years old. He was incredibly attached to her, and for the first few weeks after he came to us, he would stand by the window crying, waiting for her return. He didn't want us near him. It was heartbreaking to watch. There is so much trauma experienced by these young fostered and adopted children.

Nathan found it easier to attach to David, perhaps because David was outside of his experience, whereas I was Mummy in a whole series of other mother figures. Just knowing Nathan could make attachments was what we were looking for in those early days, so we were more than happy, even if it was just David to begin with.

From the beginning, I knew he needed help to trust, and so I would go and sit in his bedroom and say, 'I'm here if you need a hug.'

He would refuse to look at me, talk to me or go near me. So, I would just sit, sometimes for up to an hour, casually waiting. More often than not, Nathan would eventually silently reverse into me, backing into my embrace. These types of moments have kept both David and me going over the years.

Nathan behaved in the same way when he hurt himself. The shame he felt at being in pain was so huge that he could not bring himself to ask for help. The idea of having to rely on someone else was too great a risk. Instead, he would hide away. I remember the day when Nathan finally walked towards me, crying, arms out, trusting that I could hold his pain and comfort him. That feeling was incredible, and one for which I had waited for six years. From that moment, he would allow me to see his trembling lips. He cried a lot more and trusted a lot more.

Part of adoption is a lifelong commitment to walking alongside a person as they try to make sense of what has happened in their early life, and this is not always easy.

Parenting children who are different demands different ways of parenting. Initially, the biggest issue is that the rest of the world has a way of doing parenting and you are expected to follow suit. The pressure on parents to work in a particular, universally acceptable way is ever present. For those of us parenting children who are different in any way, it's impossible to stick to the norms. We cannot do things in the usual way. When we are desperately trying to find our feet, it's incredibly discouraging to face the judgement of family, friends, schools, communities and even strangers! Sometimes, that judgement can be even closer to home, with you and your partner disagreeing over parenting styles. All too often, when a parent steps into a new style, it doesn't work straight away, and so the pressure to either go back to the old ways or do something else that's new and different in an effort to solve things quickly is overwhelming. We may relent and go back to our old, traditional ways of parenting, but we soon learn that, at best, it has no impact on our child, while at worst, it can actually damage them.

At times, we have felt like hopeless failures: unable to get the results we are meant to get, unable to meet the needs of our children, unable to lead our family properly. Of course, many parents feel this pressure, but for those of us who have children with complex needs and feel like we're required to step up into super-parent mode, it can be a slow and very lonely road. We had our whole lives to think about how to build and guide a family, and now we find ourselves learning on the hoof, making snap decisions, having to think creatively, all while being physically, mentally and emotionally exhausted. We have had to be focused across four different children, all with specific different needs, and all requiring different ways of doing things. There is no one-size-fits-all here. Every day brings a new challenge we have to learn about, fully understand and try to respond well to. We have to navigate our way through acronyms and the language of health, social care and education. We are like psychotherapists living with four clients twenty-four hours a day.

Non-Violent Resistance

We have had to learn the ultra-sensitivity required to operate a push-and-pull relationship with our children, understanding when to bring pressure to bear and when to back off, what to tolerate and where there needs to be a boundary set. During Nathan's early years, we learned of a parenting method called non-violent resistance (NVR).[47] Developed in Israel by Haim Omer, it offers a non-confrontational way through conflict, but one where resistance is still brought to bear and change is sought. It can be incredibly helpful for families, schools and communities, and is now used worldwide in many contexts. For us, it provided empowerment and a regaining of parental control. Our style of parenting had entered a phase where we were passive and non-challenging until we could bear it no more, and then we would enforce a strict regime with an aggressive tone. None of this worked.

One part of NVR is that you look at all the challenging behaviours and think about them in the context of three boxes. The bottom box might be things that need looking at but aren't really a big deal. The middle box is stuff that definitely needs attention. The top box contains one behaviour you have chosen to work on with your child as a priority. This gives the family focus and allows for small wins. It also means that everyone knows what the aim is and what to do when there are other negative behaviours being presented.

If you were a visitor to our home, you may witness Nathan shout, slam a door and stomp upstairs. You may then see David and I give each other a thumbs-up. In your view a child has just totally disrespected his parents, and it looks like he's been allowed to get away with awful behaviour. To us, it may be the first time he has not been violent towards a person or thrown something, so he has actually managed to exercise self-control. All things are comparative, so Nathan walking away rather than being physically violent represents a step in the right direction, and a small win for him and us.

When Arlo first restarted school, they may have gone in with their hair unbrushed. Having spent a whole three years out of school, we were over the moon that Arlo was getting up, getting dressed and going to school. These days, Arlo wouldn't go anywhere with unbrushed hair, but what constitutes a 'win' in our world may be a whole world away from what a win would be for another family. It really helps when you know you're working to a plan. It reminds us we are on the same page, slowly moving forwards. Raising children with additional needs is a much slower process; the age markers that are routinely used to measure neurotypical children are very often not applicable. Different children will often reach the same destination by different routes at different speeds. That's OK; it's not a race.

Looking at us now, it appears that David and I are on the same page, that we shape-shifted smoothly into being super-equipped parents – but there were a lot of bumps along the way.

A lot.

Increasing Presence

We got on to the same page in the end, but finding unity within our parenting is an ongoing task. Every season throws up a new challenge, a new something you've never had to think about before, and we just have to evolve again and get our parenting shaped for the new challenge.

A major area in communication for us is the wonderful combination of 'being present' and 'holding the space'. By being present, we mean embodying the moment, sitting in it, being alert to what's happening and noticing things: reading each other's body language, facial expressions, actions and words. Being emotionally available to our children and one another is key in our family's continued growth and unity. Emotional availability helps the other person to feel safe and held. It's not always an easy stance to keep, and there are many times when we may be in the room, but we aren't available. We may be geographically present, but inside we are shut down and closed for business. When we are exhausted, this seems to be the natural response, so it's with good reason: it's self-preservation. The main thing is to be aware of our own personal headspace and to keep moving forward.

David has a good tactic if a child rushes in to tell him

something when he's on the phone. If he says, 'I can't talk now, I'm on a call,' all they'll hear is, 'I can't.' If, however he says, 'Can you give me a couple of minutes? I really want to hear what you've got to say,' they know he's listening to them and that hearing them is his priority.

Sometimes we also 'increase our presence' in very intentional ways. By this, I mean stepping into the space of the other person, but without an agenda or need to change how the person feels, get their attention, or start a conversation. Every parent wants to be able to solve the problems their child faces; it's a natural response. Over the years, I have learned solving all my children's problems for them means I am not teaching them resilience – and, in the case of mental health, all I am doing is putting pressure on them to change or perform for me. That's not healthy; in fact, it can make things worse. I have found I am of far greater help to my children when I simply make myself available.

A few years ago, when Ty was struggling with a very low mood, I remember feeling totally powerless to help him. One day, I decided to try a new approach by simply going into his bedroom and, with permission, sitting on the end of the bed. In typical teen fashion, he looked at me like I was a burden. I said I would be leaving in one minute, and one minute later he told me my time was up. I did this every day for about a week, and gradually increased the time to about five minutes. At best, Ty tolerated me, but after a week he got used to 'crazy' Mum coming into his room and just sitting in silence.

Then something began to shift.

Ty began to ask me to come in and sit in his room with him. This eventually led to him sharing how he felt. This would be the moment of a real test. Would I be able to resist telling him what would make him feel better, strategising or gee-ing him up?

I listened. I sat in the silence and nodded, acknowledging that I had heard what he was saying.

I made no suggestions. Often, I simply told him I had heard him, and that I noticed he was finding things really tough. I remember saying, 'I can't change how you feel, but I can sit alongside you in it.'

Being heard and not having to pretend he was happy was key to Ty's forward motion. When a person feels they have to mask or pretend all day in the outside world, it's vital that there is a space somewhere where they can just be themselves and be permitted to express a whole range of emotions, both positive and negative.

The Communication Model

This massive period of evolution of us as parents was also when David and I learned about the communication model. This precious strategy has changed the way all of us get through conversation, and especially conflict. We repeat back what the person has said. Quite literally, word for word, without judgement. This gives the person time to reshape thinking and, where necessary, rephrase hurtful or harmful words towards themselves or others.

There is something we used to hear from Arlo all the time in the playground line-up for class in the morning: 'I don't want to go into school. The work's too hard and the teacher hates me.'

Initially, we would have said, 'The teacher doesn't hate you. She said just the other day that she loves the way you work in class, and she can help you with the harder work – that's what she's there for. You'll be fine once you're in there.'

We imagined this would be reassuring. We were correcting wrong ideas, and paving the way to a smooth day for our child. Or so we thought.

In truth, it invalidated the overwhelming sense of anxiety our child was feeling, which then led to a bit of a scene in the playground. In time, we realised a completely counter-intuitive response was more effective.

'I don't want to go into school. The work's too hard and the teacher hates me.'

'I hear you. You don't want to go into school. The work's too hard and the teacher hates you.'

'Yes,' came the reply, followed by our child walking straight into class, quite content.

Arlo just needed to be heard and to have their feelings validated.

Sometimes, repeating back allows the person to reflect on whether what they are saying is true or kind or necessary. It helps the person to de-escalate, correct themselves or shape what they really think and feel.

It is also helpful to slow things down. Not all of us process communication at superhighway speeds. By slowing down the conversation and allowing for moments of silence, we make way for more reasoned thinking.

Broadening Language

Language is another area that we have found to be important. We encourage one another to use a broader spectrum of words. Social media majors in absolutes and catastrophic language, so words like abuser, control, narcissist, trauma, gaslighting and depression are bandied about for everyday use, in everyday situations. This not only escalates conflict but also devalues the experience of those who are encountering situations these words truly describe. Some sadness can be a normal part of life; that is different to depression or despair. Asking your child to do something does not make you a narcissist. Someone shouting doesn't instantly make them an abuser. We try to increase our emotional vocabulary and sharpen our understanding of what words mean so that we can be concise and accurate in our communication.

In all the tests our children have undergone, the results have shown that every child has a vocabulary way beyond their years. And yet if I ask Tylan or Arlo how they feel, they will, invariably, say, 'I'm fine.'

For them, 'fine' can mean anything from ecstatic to feeling very low – or hot or cold or anxious or calm. If a child says they are fine when they are not, but we haven't noticed, we will then be shocked when they melt down, so it's important to gauge the real meaning of words in order to understand exactly how people are feeling and the scale of those feelings.

When they were younger, we often used Dr Tony Attwood's CAT Kit,[48] a communication tool that has many pages dedicated to emotions. For example, a page for the word 'happy' will have twenty Velcro emoji faces with different words underneath, each portraying a more nuanced word and expression, such as joyful, cheeky or content. This stretching of linguistic expression has helped our children to expand their emotional vocabulary and also connect with how they are feeling in that moment. Sometimes, one of the cartoon facial expressions itself will represent more than the word for them. We have increased our non-verbal skills in order to enter our children's worlds. Paying attention to their body language, facial expressions and breathing, and noticing when they may be disinclined to eat or wash or sleep, or when they seem to be disengaged with their self-care or even with the things they usually enjoy, can give us clues as to what might be going on for them on the inside.

Consent

Another part of communication that has become highlighted over the past few years is consent. Modelling consent should be fundamental to our parenting experience. When a child is never allowed an opinion and never allowed to decline a request, that request is then interpreted as a demand, and their world is read as a place in which they have no agency. Consequently, it is likely they will grow into under-confident adults, unable to state an opinion, say what they like or dislike, or say no when they are uncomfortable. When we don't allow our children to refuse us, when we never back down, we are fostering an atmosphere of people-pleasing that doesn't serve them well as they grow older. Hear me on this: I'm not saying encourage your child to rebel, but allowing them to have preferences and moments when they want their opinion respected is vitally important. Not having to hug every relative or be made to speak on the phone or being permitted to have different political or faith views to their parents, matters.

Demand Avoidance and Anxiety

Children who are anxious, for whatever reason, will normally have some level of demand avoidance. This may not present in outright refusal; it may be that a child makes it impossible to do something by saying they are unwell, they can't face the teacher, they are tired or they cannot manage. While all of these things may be true, it's important to find out why they are reluctant to participate in certain activities. Anxiety is often sitting at the root of the problem.

When someone experiences high levels of anxiety, their toleration levels decrease, and adding a further demand can prove to be impossible. We have sometimes noticed that activities our children are more than able to do one week are suddenly impossible the next. This used to confound us, but as we began to explore anxiety and how it was impacting each of our children, we started to see patterns. There was a relational, triangular cycle occurring between anxiety, toleration and demand. Each was connected to the other, but anxiety was the driver.

We experience anxiety for any number of reasons, but if we feel heard, understood and accepted, it can have an immediate and positive effect. This is the single biggest argument for meeting the needs of a child in school (or in the workplace) and making what are known as reasonable adjustments. These small adjustments let the person know they are being seen and considered, and this alone, as much as the actual adjustment itself, can help with reducing anxiety.

It is believed that some autistic people have what's called pathological demand avoidance (PDA) as part of their autism profile. The word pathological simply means 'outside of the normal range of what would be expected'. Although avoiding demands is something we all do from time to time, in the case of PDA, the demand avoidance can be all-encompassing. Here are the traits of PDA:[49]

- resists and avoids the ordinary demands of life
- uses social strategies as part of avoidance: for example, distracting, giving excuses
- appears sociable, but lacks some understanding
- experiences excessive mood swings and impulsivity
- appears comfortable in role play and pretence
- displays obsessive behaviour that is often focused on other people

Both Arlo and Nathan have very high levels of demand avoidance, Arlo because of their autism and Nathan because adherence equates to trust, and trust is tricky for him.

With Arlo, we have found giving choices rather than making demands is the best way to communicate. 'It's time to get ready for bed now,' has become, 'I've popped the blue and the red pyjamas at the end of your bed.' Arlo will then perceive this as a choice rather than a demand. We have learned the push and pull of negotiation. If we push too hard, Arlo may shut down and become totally non-compliant, even to the detriment of their own desires. They may have an event they are super-excited about going to. They are running late. We hurry them along, saying, 'Quickly, get your shoes on, sweetie.'

Mistake.

Arlo will then say, 'OK, I'm not going, and it's because of you. I was going to go, but now you're making me, so I'm not going.'

What we say next will determine the day's outcome. We could say, 'OK, no problem. It's your choice; don't go.' Usually, this would get us nowhere, as Arlo will simply escalate into shouting. We have found it's better to say, 'Sorry I was rushing you. I know you really want to get to the event. We'll go when you're ready.'

This may mean they miss the event, but there is every chance they will get out of the house sooner if they are encouraged to be calm, and that involves us de-escalating. We are really aware that even when they are excited about going somewhere, it will invariably involve desperately high levels of anxiety, so the main focus is not on compliance but calmness.

Nathan's demand avoidance comes from a very different angle. Having to make a choice or a decision can prove to be very hard for Nathan. This is because all the early life decisions that were made by others on his behalf, although well meaning, had what could be perceived by Nathan as catastrophic consequences. As a result of this, he could treat even the most mundane decision as though it carried the potential for disaster. He would constantly suffer from choice fatigue, which would result in him making a choice, only to change his mind and angrily blame us for placing him in the impossible situation of having to state a preference. It seemed as though Nathan was non-compliant and even defiant, but it was with good reason. When Nathan first came to us at two years old, I would sit him in the highchair in the morning and give him a bowl of cornflakes. He would push the bowl away, sometimes tipping it over the edge, spilling the milk all over the floor, and say, 'No want it.'

I learned very quickly not to put the milk in until he had made a choice.

I would tip the cornflakes back in the box and pour out some Rice Krispies.

'No want it.'

He would then point to the cornflakes.

I would re-pour the cornflakes.

'No want it.'

And round we would go in circles.

My old style of parenting would lead me to say, 'Well, this is your breakfast, and this is all you're getting.' And sometimes that would work. At other times, I would be ducking as the bowl flew towards my face.

We have had to learn to be negotiating ninjas. Traditional parenting says that consistency works; just keep doing the same thing over and over, and eventually your child will conform. We aren't in disagreement with that. Except that our children are different, and any parent who has children like ours will let you know that often, it doesn't work. Nathan could sit for hours in the highchair, not eating. Remember, an adopted child may be a child who has experienced being left for hours unfed, unwashed, unheld. In a proverbial staring competition, it's likely that this child will win. Some mornings with Nathan were impossible; I would have to get him out to an activity or go out to work myself, so time became a factor. Letting your child go out without breakfast is also an absolute no-no, so often we found ourselves with a real parenting challenge.

Eventually, we found a natural form-and-flow style of doing things in these situations. 'Form' is where you have a plan, and you are going to try everything you can to stick to the plan and hold your ground. Holding your resistance is important. 'Flow' informs you that there is more than one way of doing things, and sometimes compromise is better: finding a middle ground. In the case of the breakfast cereal, I would simply leave two bowls of cereal, both with milk in, on his highchair tray and leave the room.

Alone and unobserved, Nathan could decide without defaulting to a choice-crisis. He would happily eat one of the breakfasts. As soon as he had started, I would re-enter the kitchen, praise him for making a good decision, and simply pour away the other cereal (wasteful, I know). I would have to get in quick, as Nathan would also try to eat both bowls. At every meal, Nathan would stuff any and every morsel of food available into his mouth. Fearful of not being fed, he would sometimes eat until he threw up. It's truly dreadful what even a few weeks of early-life trauma or neglect can do to us.

For many children who are fostered and adopted, at the root of many of the issues like this is a huge underlying sense of shame: a deeply held belief that one is not good enough, a sense of having to carry rejection and humiliation. Shame has absolutely no earthly use. It is like the appendix of the mind. Having a sense of wrongdoing and taking responsibility when we make wrong choices or perform harmful actions is good, but shame will have you lost down a rabbit hole of self-loathing, unravelling any positive feelings you have towards yourself. This is the area we have had to work on with Nathan. He doesn't have the secure inner scaffolding like our other children, so we have to shore him up – and it's late in the day. The foundations that should have been there from birth are missing, so building his self-esteem has become an underpinning job, as we seek to help him to value himself and understand his significance and his place in the world. Those early weeks, months and years set a trajectory that is very hard to shift once it's in place.

Yes Versus No

Scientific studies show that the word 'no' causes a negative response in our brains. A 2007 report revealed:

> No and Yes were associated with opposite brain-behaviour responses; while No was negatively valenced, produced slower response times, and evoked a negative signal in the right lateral orbitofrontal cortex (OFC), Yes was positively valenced, produced faster response times and evoked a positive signal in a contiguous region of the OFC.[50]

With all children, a straight 'no' can elicit an adverse response. In the 'terrible twos' phase, parents know all too well the impact of the word 'no' on their child. For most children, the word 'no', although unwelcome, begins to carry less weight and there are fewer challenges as they age. With children who have any form of demand avoidance, however, these adverse reactions continue. Demand avoidance may have its roots in being neurodivergent or having experienced early life trauma. The reactions may come in the form of tantrums, meltdowns, shouting, crying, door slamming, etc. No child wants to hear the answer 'no' to something they really want. But for most of us, 'no', 'don't', 'can't' and 'shouldn't' are staples of our vocabulary. These words aren't just used in response to requests, but also to steer children away from danger and towards good and safe behaviours.

Although the word 'no' is important in the setting of

boundaries and equipping our children with the tools they need to deal with the real world, using negatives too often can shut down a child's initiative and cause them to think inside the box. Saying 'no' less frequently can make a positive difference. Being spoken to positively instead of constantly being told what's not on offer helps children develop problem-solving and critical-thinking skills. It also points them towards positives rather than just stating negatives.

If overused, children can become immune to the word 'no'; we devalue its currency. I've lost count of the times early on in my parenting journey when our children would start a sentence, 'I know you're going to say no, but . . .' because I would often say 'no' without explaining why or giving alternatives.

Explaining *why* the answer is 'no' helps children to learn to make better choices.

Giving a child an alternative or a different option distracts the child away from the thing you don't want them to do or have.

The sting of the word 'no' can be replaced with:

'I think we can probably do that later . . .'

'I understand why you would want this thing, however . . .'

'I can see you really like that . . .'

'I can see you're really struggling to think about something else right now . . .'

We went from saying, 'No, I am not buying that,' to, 'I can see you really like that, and I understand why – it looks really nice – but that's not why we are here, so maybe we can look at it another day.'

When Tylan was little, we moved our language from a straight 'no' to encompass this more nuanced language. The issue for Ty was that he would become hyper-focused on getting something. We would answer: 'Maybe we can do/get that later.'

Ty worked out that this 'later' thing took some time, so created a phrase that calmed his impulsive desires. 'Is that after later?' he would ask, trying to work out how long things would take.

'Yes!' we would reply.

The idea of 'after later' gave Ty the time to decompress and shift the hyper-focus. The thing that was so desired in the moment became less of a deal-breaker if there was the potential for 'after later'.

As a parent, it's easy to feel like we are directing, bossing and nagging our children the whole time. Finding simple ways of reframing our language can really make a difference.

The Importance of Praise

Back in 2019, I was asked to film a feature for the BBC's *The One Show* on the work of leading child psychologist Sue Westwood and her team at De Montfort University.[51] They had been looking at the impact of praise upon our children, and had launched an initiative to encourage parents to praise their children at least five times a day, but with an emphasis on the best *ways* to praise.[52] When I think of how David and I praise, I think we perhaps used to drown our children in the stuff, and it has really helped David and me to take stock. Here is our brief summary of the main points of the initiative, but I encourage you to delve deeper, as we found it incredibly helpful.

Increase the number of times you praise your children by

looking out for when they do something good. The idea is to 'catch them' being good and ensuring that you comment.

Describe exactly what you are happy about. Being specific can help our children to understand more clearly what it is we are pleased with or impressed by. This helps them to repeat the action. If our praise is too vague, they have no idea what it is they have done right. For instance, in the past we may have said, 'Your behaviour at Molly's house was outstanding, well done. We are so pleased with you.'

Now, we would say 'We noticed how well you played when you were with Molly today. You shared the toys and took turns well. We are so pleased with you.'

It's subtle but significant.

Similarly, I think in the past, if one of the kids did a good painting, we would tell them they were the next Picasso; that they were world class, the best thing we'd ever seen. As lovely as this appeared, we realised it wasn't necessarily helpful. How do they repeat the action? What if their next painting wasn't as good? We realised it was better to point out the things we liked about the painting, telling them we loved the way they'd made the sun look like it was shining by adding some rays to it, or that we loved the way they'd mixed the paints to get a particular colour. With this type of praise, our children had a measurable indicator of what they had achieved and what constituted 'good' work.

Praise effort rather than ability or achievement. This is such an important area for children with additional needs. If the focus is on effort, then it allows us to praise our children for all the trying they are doing, whether it's leading to measurable success or not.

Look for little changes. Don't wait for them to do

something perfectly before giving them recognition. Celebrating the small wins is the best way forward. Just before lockdown, I felt that my parenting efforts were netting absolutely no results. I was discouraged. I decided to start a 'small wins' journal. I would write down any good feelings I was experiencing in my parenting, and I would also note down anything positive the children had done. Within a few days, I had pages of writing. It was a good reminder that positive things are happening all the time: things that it is essential not to miss.

Therapy

There are many types of therapy out there. Some work for our children, while others don't. The truth is, accessing these therapies in a timely manner is just about impossible unless you can pay vast sums of money. Post-Covid, some of these services have even closed their books to new clients.

Talking therapies include cognitive behavioural therapy (CBT)[53] and dialectical behavioural therapy (DBT).[54] Generally speaking, CBT looks at negative thinking that traps a person in a vicious cycle. It looks at current problems (as opposed to historical) and how to break them down into manageable parts. DBT looks at holding two opposing thoughts, accepting oneself and changing behaviours.

Trauma therapy[55] can be super-helpful for our children who have had negative experiences in early life, or at school or home. There are various ways in which this therapy is applied. It may involve CBT or DBT, but may also include eye movement desensitisation reprocessing (EMDR).[56] This is where the patient is encouraged to think of a negative memory while the therapist applies bi-lateral stimulation (typically eye movements), which has the impact of lessening the evocative images and softening the memories. Somatic therapy[57] focuses on the physical impact of negative emotions and trauma found in the body. If you like, the headline is the story of what happened, the feelings are the emotional responses to what happened, and the somatic part is the sensations that are physically felt in the body.

Integrated therapy is often helpful for our complex children. This is where a therapist draws from several therapeutic practices and tailors the therapy to suit the client. There are also dance or art or Lego therapies, all of which can be incredibly helpful for children who want to steer away from face-to-face talking. Then there is Theraplay.[58] This is used for younger children, allowing them to lead play so that they can recover a sense of agency and control.

It's well worth finding out how each of these therapies work, and what's available in your area. If you are accessing help from your local authority, everything they offer can be found on the local authority website under 'Local Offer'. This will also include the Special Educational Needs support available in your area.

There are hundreds of therapies and strategies out there, with new data and ideas emerging constantly. Finding what works for you and your child can take time. Also, what works one week may not the next, or what didn't work before may now work well. As parents, we never stop shape-shifting.

Medication

Not everyone chooses to proceed down the medication route, and that is perfectly OK. It's certainly not always necessary. On occasions with our children, we have found medication to be quite literally a lifesaver. One thing to consider is the length of time it can take to get the medication right. It seems that mental health medication is less of an exact science than taking meds to meet our physical needs. It would be great to remove the stigma from choosing this pathway, but equally we must, as with any medication, be aware of the long-term side effects.

As of now, Olive has chosen not to take ADHD medication, as they tried about six different types and none of them seemed to work without horrid side effects. Olive also says they need their hyperactivity in order to perform their acting the way they do. Nathan, on the other hand, needs his ADHD meds to get any level of sustained focus. As you can see, it's an individual thing.

The best advice here is to join parent groups where you can ask questions and make a considered choice. This goes for just about all of the subjects in this book. You can find these online (mainly through Facebook). Again, there should also be information on your local authority's website under 'Local Offer'. There are also several parent carer forums all over the UK.[59]

School Adjustments

There are so many small adjustments that can be made to make life for our children tolerable, manageable, positive and even fun. The biggest adjustment is in the minds of those who encounter our children. If this mindset is right, then it is likely everything else our children need will follow. Communication between school and home is vital if we desire a healthy and happy experience for our children. This can take time and hard work, but it can be achieved – and we really see the benefit to the child.

Lunch Pass

Sometimes, autistic children or those with sensory needs struggle with the area of eating. Busy, noisy canteens, squashed seating and people breathing – or, even worse, talking – over food can be problematic. A lunch pass allows a child to take a friend into the lunch area before anyone else arrives, thereby limiting these challenges.

Seating

Where a child sits in class can impact them, so seating is something to consider. The visual distractions of the room may be harder when a child sits further back in the room. Sitting with a friend may help neurodivergent children.

An 'I Need to Leave the Room' Card

Children may benefit from an 'I need to leave the room' card, which has one blue side and one yellow side. The child can place it on their desk: blue side up means they are fine, yellow side up means they need to get out. The teacher can then respond accordingly.

Homework

Working out the best strategy around homework should be discussed with the school, parents and child. Sometimes children love homework, but quite often, school can be so traumatising that the concept of continuing work at home can make the child feel as though school never ends. If we want to keep the home a low-anxiety zone, it may be better to work out how the child can complete homework in school, or, if appropriate (in primary school), whether they can not have homework.

Detention and aggressive communication

Similarly, detention or even the threat of detention can make our children not want to go to school. A teacher shouting at the whole class may be experienced by the autistic child as the teacher shouting at them in particular. Our children will need reassurance. When a child has a social communication issue, full explanation may be necessary so that they understand exactly what you mean. Otherwise, they may fill in the gaps and come to a wrong conclusion.

Exams

Exam conditions can be tailored so that the student has their own space during examinations, and timings can be extended so that the child has the extra time necessary to process the tasks set before them.

School Uniform

School uniform, with its itchy labels, can be incredibly challenging for those with sensory issues, as can feeling too hot or too cold. There should be allowances made for children who struggle with sensory processing. Removing a blazer in class is hardly an act of outright rebellion! I would also love to see a time when schools don't sweat the small stuff regarding uniform, hair and jewellery.

Mentors

Having mentors or a buddy system can be so helpful for children who struggle with finding friends. All too often, you will find the SEND (Special Educational Needs and Disability) child alone in the playground, without friends but often desperate to join in. Schemes like this also help the mentor/buddy children to develop empathy and inclusion.

Safe People and Safe Spaces

In secondary school, a child may need to understand who their safe people are: the teachers to whom they can turn if they are feeling anxious or worried. We used to have a list of them for Tylan. A list like this should also include safe spaces, places within the school where the child can go to be alone or sit quietly.

Learning Breaks

Learning breaks should be written into the school schedule for SEN children. Regular breaks help them to self-regulate, refocus and reset. Sometimes a physical activity during a break can aid this process.

The Blurt Box

Using a 'blurt box' can help children who want to speak constantly or who, like Arlo, want to give a running commentary on what's happening in class and how well (or badly!) the teacher is teaching. A blurt box is a little box into which notes can be posted by the child. At the end of each session, a teaching assistant can go through it and address any thoughts that may be troubling the child. Arlo found this very helpful in primary school.

Dropping Non-Essential Subjects

Another area that really helped all our children was dropping non-essential subjects that they found stressful, such as learning a foreign language, as this is something that can be returned to in later life, post-school. We want our children to learn as much as possible in school, of course, and most children will manage the curriculum. But some won't, and for these children, adjustments like this can make a real difference.

Four key areas to consider inside the classroom are:

- What is the sensory environment like? Does the room smell? Is it noisy or crowded? Even squeaky doors can be very difficult for children to block out, so a classroom at the end of a corridor where there is a constant thoroughfare of students can be problematic for those with sensory issues.
- How is the child's relationship to the subject? If every Wednesday afternoon they are melting down, it could be that the subject they have every Wednesday afternoon is the cause.
- How is the child's relationship with others in the class? This is particularly important in secondary school, when some children dread certain classes because of their classmates.
- How is the child's relationship with the teacher? With our children, we have found the more they know a teacher likes them, the more settled they will be. Being accepted and understood means the world to our children.

As we learn about a child, we learn what works for them, how they communicate best and how we can help them to interpret the world around them. We can also help the world to understand a particular child; we advocate for them and hopefully help them to advocate for themselves. The ideas we have listed above are really a starting block to get you thinking. You will come up with dozens more that are specific to your child and their needs once you get started.

DAVID

As vocal coaches, we have always had a three-tier strategy, and it's also a good structure for our parenting journey: train, coach, maintain.

Train

Training is teaching a skill or type of behaviour that is previously unknown by the learner; a common example would be potty training. A toddler has no concept of how to use a potty until taught. It's not a natural process; like most things in life, it's learned behaviour. At the earliest developmental stage, a child is like a sponge. Everything is new, everything is unfamiliar, and at this stage of learning, our responsibility and our objective as parents or carers is to equip our charges with the necessary skills to begin navigating life. Talent is natural, but the development of talent and the mastering of skills require teaching, application, repetition and time. When it comes to time, the pace of teaching can differ from child to child.

We know from our experience as vocal coaches that

people learn at different paces and in different ways. With neurotypical (NT) children, the pace at which they learn and recall, and their styles of learning, are likely to be different from those of neurodivergent (ND) children. It's essential that we avoid comparisons. Each child will present us with a unique teaching opportunity and carry their own unique learning challenges. There will almost certainly be areas where they move seamlessly from teaching to coaching to maintenance, while in others they appear to remain perpetually in the teaching bracket. The child that is completely toilet-trained, has impeccable table manners and makes their bed each morning may have to be reminded every day to brush their teeth.

It is normal that a child will leap forward, moving seamlessly through the stages in some areas and yet getting stuck in others. I've learned the hard way that consistent, patient encouragement is needed. My tried-and-trusted 'How many times do I have to tell you?' and, 'Do I have to say the same thing every day?' did not have the desired effect. What I did learn was that how we teach at the earliest developmental stages can have a lifelong effect on that child's relationship with learning. Therefore, recognising the small wins is a much more effective way of gradually eliciting change and easing the graduation from teaching into coaching.

Children who are different in any way also have the added challenge of trying to work out where they fit in the world; school can be traumatic, and a child's headspace may already be at capacity just trying to work it all out. Some things that come easily to a NT child may take years of repeated learning to master for ND children.

Coach

Coaching works on the basis that the one being coached at least loosely knows what they are doing. The job of the coach is to enable them to do it better, by working alongside them, and giving tips and strategies that help to aid how well a task is done. If it's cooking, for example, the child will perform the action and the coach will be on hand to answer questions and offer advice. It's very tempting during this stage to step in, as the child might take an age to do something that you could accomplish in seconds, but it's essential to stay present without interfering.

Once, as a teenager, I told my sixty-something grandmother that, because she was 'so old', I could do something twice as fast as she could. Her response was that 'if' indeed I could do it at twice the speed, I would still finish a little *after* her, as she could do it with less than half the effort. I didn't believe her, and asked her to talk me through how the task could be done with 'less than half the effort'. She explained, and she was right: my wise old gran got the same thing done in less than half the time, even though I was working faster. I didn't realise it then, but she was coaching me. I knew 'how to', but she knew a better, more efficient way.

A parent coaching a child is different to a tennis or football coach working with an athlete, as sometimes we have to coach by stealth. Because the emotions involved in any family can make it much harder for your child to listen to you than to a relative stranger, coaching can sometimes feel frustrating and discouraging. These are the times when we have to trust that if our words go unheard or unheeded, our example is still silently read and observed. There is a quote often attributed to

Mark Twain: 'When I was a boy of fourteen, my father was so ignorant I could hardly stand to have the old man around. But when I got to be twenty-one, I was astonished at how much the old man had learned in seven years.'

The ones we are coaching can be so self-assuredly unaware of the mistakes they are making that correcting, advising and coaching can sometimes feel impossible. If this is you, stay present, keep on living rather than giving examples, and don't give up hope. This stage will pass and the wisdom of what you are modelling will be seen – even if, as in the quote above, your children think it's you who has done all the changing.

Maintain

Unlike the other stages, maintaining, as defined here, isn't task- or performance-based. It is much more about character, and the people our children are evolving into. It's about providing a true north towards which they can navigate, and a safe space where they can have their personhood and identity endorsed and affirmed.

This stage can only begin when there is respect and maturity in the relationship. Carrie and I are really adamant (particularly as children of single parents) that our children remain children and do not have the weight of our world on their shoulders from an early age.

This transition into a more mature, equal relationship can be a confusing time for parents, as we inevitably have to redefine our parenting identities and recalibrate our parent–child relationship. Conversely, it can be a glorious time of beginning a new stage of a relationship with a fully formed adult who's just beginning to take flight on wings that you have taught them how to spread.

If our child becomes our friend too soon, we can inadvertently place heavy burdens and expectations on them. Sometimes loneliness, or a lack of someone to share with, can make the temptation to bring our children into our confidence irresistible. But if their shoulders are not yet broad enough to carry the weight that we need to unload, we can unintentionally cause damage.

For the health of your relationship with your child and their emotional well-being, it's essential to know which stage they are in.

Some parents have the opposite problem; their child has grown up in front of them and they haven't fully noticed. I fell squarely into that category with our eldest. In fact, most of the verbal miscommunications and disconnections of my parenting journey have been as a result of failing to recognise when the child I am talking to is not in the stage I am attributing to them. Speaking to a fifteen-year-old as though they were ten is a sure-fire recipe for misunderstanding.

When Olive, our eldest child, was in their early twenties I would often filter the concerns they shared with me through my own worldview and my core values, which didn't always chime with theirs. They, as a twenty-two-year-old, would be having an adult conversation with me, and I would be speaking to them as though they were still seventeen. I found it hard to distinguish between being a listening ear and insisting on offering what, in my opinion, was the solution. It took a while before I fully grasped that they needed me to be collaborative, not prescriptive. I would then be offended when they were more inclined to share with Carrie and not with me. The reason Olive found it easier to share with Carrie was because she had realised earlier than I did that although Olive was *our* child, they were no longer *a* child.

When our adult children share themselves with us, when they speak of identity, sexuality, gender, relationships, life decisions and other big issues, they are not demanding that we mirror them, or become like them. As a parent, there comes a point where we must stop demanding the same of them.

Whichever stage our children are in – whether teach, coach or maintain – we try to be prepared to meet them where they are, and to offer help when it's required, advice when it's requested and, eventually, friendship.

What we are learning along the way

1. There are many ways to communicate, not all of which are verbal.
2. Our parenting is constantly evolving and new strategies are coming through all the time.
3. Little adjustments can cost nothing but have a powerful impact.

Questions for the reader to consider

1. In what areas of your communication do you have room for improvement?
2. How aware are you of non-verbal communication?
3. What strategies, here or otherwise, may work for your child?

6

RESILIENCE

CARRIE

At the age of twenty, after two years of illness and countless tests, I was diagnosed with Crohn's disease. Being diagnosed with a life-changing and incurable disease was devastating. The treatments and exploratory tests were brutal. By the age of twenty-three, soon after I married David, I was very ill, and spent nearly a year in and out of hospital. I had major surgery to remove a section of my bowel. Suddenly, my identity became 'sick person'. This was not what I had planned for my life. I had set my goals and boundaries; I had things I wanted to achieve, and areas of life I vowed I would never go back to, having had a very difficult childhood.

Sickness was off my radar. I had everything worked out. But this was something I had never made headspace for.

Often, major issues have multiple layers, battles happening concurrently, and these things can challenge or change our views of ourselves and our futures. The double battle occurring for me was within my body and my mindset. I questioned what I was here for; what was my purpose as a sick person? My life was now one of living in and out of a hospital bed. I didn't know if I would be able to have children, or if I would ever work again. I felt as though my life had been destroyed. My world became smaller and smaller until my daily existence was simply counting sixty-second instalments, just to get myself through the next hour and towards the next dose of pain-relief medication. It was a shrunken place; my life became one of toleration. It went on for months and into years.

One night, as I lay in the hospital bed, lost in isolation and confusion, the elderly lady in the bed next to mine passed away. I was in the darkest place; my dreams and aspirations had disappeared. But in that reduced place, in the depths of despair, something happened. Something within me began to shift. A new feeling started to emerge. It was not resentment, regret, or disappointment.

It was hope.

It didn't even make sense, but I could not fight its onset. Hope was being birthed in me. And then came a sentence: 'Stop looking at what you've lost and start looking at what you have left.'

The phrase kept running through my head as if on a loop. This revelation set me free. It was the life-giving moment I had hoped and prayed and longed for. My circumstances may have been the same, but I was changing. This difficult situation was bringing new life. If I only had a short life, I would make it count. If I couldn't leave my bed, then I would still find ways of creating something beautiful with my life. I sewed beautiful tapestries, I wrote letters to friends, I wrote songs; my early songwriting started there. I would offer hope to those around me and encourage other families who had members with Crohn's disease. Out of the dark place, I learned meaning-making. I found purpose. If on some days, it just didn't work out, that was OK. But the minute the pain levels decreased, I would be up, I would be productive, I would not lose hope. Timing is everything, and I do believe the day before, I wouldn't have found this hope. It came at the right moment in my journey. These things cannot be rushed. The time in the dark place is valuable, but it does not have the last word. I have found there to be a moment in every dark place that offers an opportunity to get up again and begin the walk of life.

This is a story of resilience, but it is also a story of surrender, and that surrender led to character growth beyond measure. It changed my identity, my worldview, and my purpose. What would I do with what I had left? The person who has faced their own mortality has an opportunity to live life in a more fearless and meaningful way.

At the time, I didn't think I could go through anything worse than this; I believed this would be the biggest and last test of my life! Oh, how naive I was. I remember my mother sitting by my hospital bed, telling me she wished she could take this illness for me; she would have given anything to stop my suffering. And this is how we are as parents. We would do anything to protect our children from the cruelties of this world, from the suffering and pain. Sometimes, I feel as though my life is spent running ahead of my child's arrival, preparing the way, moving and shifting everything I can to make the path as smooth as possible, taking down prejudices and challenging systems. But they still get hurt, they still get caught, they are still subject to a society that is not ready for them.

We so desperately want to make life good for our children, but we need supreme levels of patience when parenting the children we have. It would be so good to be able to just follow a step-by-step guidebook and get predictable outcomes, but that is not our family. When a child is traumatised, it makes things even harder than they already are. So far, our main aim has been to protect our children from the trauma that has happened in school.

2017

The year 2017 was one we will never forget.

Arlo, who was then eleven, went to an autism school. They had been in mainstream education up to that point, and it had worked well until the last year of primary school, when it became clear that Arlo wasn't managing so well. They wanted to walk out of class, to comment on the quality of the teaching and sometimes to disrupt the learning of other students. What should schools do in this situation? It's very difficult, because the way schools are set up means children like ours will inevitably fail. Things got so hard for Arlo's school that they suggested Arlo stayed out of school in the afternoons until, for three days in a row, they could achieve three out of five practices from a list the school had made. If Arlo could achieve this, they could attend the afternoon sessions again.

This flipped the day for David and me, who now had a child out of school in the afternoons. It made it difficult to work. The list the school had made included things like 'no blurting', 'no walking out' and 'listen to the teacher'. Arlo had a one-to-one teaching assistant (TA) with them all day, so they were supervised throughout. A child who is autistic may blurt – it's often part of the autism profile. A child with autism and ADHD may need regular learning breaks, so genuinely need to step out of class, and they may also really struggle to listen to the teacher for any length of time. So, as you can see, fulfilling the school's targets would be impossible, because our child was expected to suppress behaviours that are traits of their neurodivergence. The school had inadvertently set them up to fail. This list would prove to be impossible to achieve, and what was intended to be a few afternoons off school turned into a month; Arlo just couldn't manage to do three things three days in a row. Eventually, there came a day when Tylan went back on to suicide watch in hospital. I was unable to pick up Arlo, and so the school allowed Arlo back in.

In the autumn of 2017, when it came to deciding on a secondary school, we thought the best thing would be for Arlo to go to an autism school. We really believed it would be the dream school. In the final year of primary school, Arlo had taken to wearing a coat and hat all day. The hat even stayed on at night. When we visited the new school with Arlo, it was a hot day and they were, as ever, wearing their coat and hat. No mention was made of it by the new school staff; no one batted an eyelid. *Bingo,* we thought. *At last, somewhere that gets it, a safe space for our autistic child.* However, months later, when Arlo arrived at the new school, they were immediately told they would have to take off their coat and hat. This was equivalent to asking Arlo to walk into school naked. On top of this, the autism profile of the girls in the school was very quiet and under the radar. Some had been bullied in mainstream schools; for them, it was meant to be a safe haven after the madness of mainstream schooling. Arlo wasn't having any of it. They would sit in the class and bang the desk and shout at the top of their voice, 'Oh, we're all a bit anxious in here, aren't we?'

Arlo would be asked to leave the class, which they would refuse to do, and then all the other children had to leave the class. As you can imagine, it must have been very challenging for the school. The school's solution was to have Arlo alone in the pavilion room on the school field for the entire day – away from their new friends, with one teacher, unable to leave – for six hours a day.

One day in October 2017, I was flying to Ireland for *The One Show*. Just before the flight took off, the announcement came to switch our phones to airplane mode. I reached for my phone and saw there were multiple texts.

'Mum, I've locked myself in the toilet.'

'I can't do this any more.'

'They won't let me out of the room.'

'Please come and get me.'

'COME AND GET ME!!!'

The airplane began taxi-ing down the runway for take-off. I kept reading.

'Please, Mum, please answer, come and get me.'

'Please.'

'Please.'

'Please.'

'Please.'

'Please.'

'Please.'

'I can't do this any more.'

I switched off my phone.

It was the longest flight of my life.

A week later, Arlo was permanently excluded from the school. Now Arlo had no school.

Arlo was eleven years old and suddenly had no friends, no school, no future. The local authority sent a teacher over to our home to do some work with Arlo, but Arlo would not leave their bedroom. They were depressed and alone; their only company was me and David.

Tylan was also really struggling at this time. David and I had decided a couple of years before that the only way we could financially survive this period with our children was to job-share our time. We pretty much stopped working together; we let go of dreams and abandoned our career plans and visions of the future. The only thing we could think of, day and night, was our children and finding a way through for them. We had become full-time carers.

By this time, Ty had been on and off suicide watch for two and a half years, and had missed a huge amount of school. When your child has needs that are beyond the range of normal special needs provision (whatever that constitutes) the school or the parent can apply for an Education and Health Care Plan (EHCP). These things are like gold dust. The local authorities will sometimes do everything in their power to stop parents from getting an EHCP. They will often automatically turn down the first application, knowing that most parents won't have the money or mental resources to take it to a tribunal. Many an EHCP has been given agreement and delivered just days before the tribunal date.

The EHCP. The full, professional, detailed account of your child, their needs and what must be done to accommodate those needs.

Your child's golden ticket to a proper education.

Except that it isn't.

The EHCP is not worth the paper it's written on if it is not applied properly or doesn't match the child's ever-changing needs. A child that may have started out needing a few adjustments and some extra attention may require totally different adjustments if they are now suicidal, being bullied and missing large chunks of school. If your child experiences psychosis, hears voices or sees things that aren't there, then what they need in school at thirteen is not what was arranged when they were nine. If your child is self-harming or has developed an eating disorder, the adjustments must change. As parents, we are usually left to seek out the most compassionate person we can find in school and plead our child's case. The EHCP has an annual review, but often this only allows for minor adaptations.

Trying to get the school to work with you can be terribly difficult. There are schools who are incredible and respectful and accommodating, and there are schools whose priority simply isn't SEND. With the thousands of SEND parents we have spoken to over the years, we have found most (not all) of the mainstream school experiences of collaboration to be sadly lacking. Sometimes they have been obstructive; sometimes they have shown reluctance to accommodate even the things that cost nothing. It's really about mindset. It's very hard to get people with fixed mindsets to shift their thinking. When schools 'get it', however, it's a joy to collaborate.

Back in 2016, after Ty had been sent multiple messages from bullies telling him to kill himself, I remember asking the school if they would do a piece of work on restorative justice, as we believed that simply giving kids a fixed exclusion would not change behaviours. I was refused. The two girls had been given a week off school. They were told that upon their return to school, they must not approach Tylan or speak to him.

Kids are clever. Kids can be mean.

The girls would walk past Ty and suddenly stamp hard on the ground, burst out laughing or make a loud noise as they went past. If Ty was in the playground speaking to a friend, they would come up and speak to that same friend, while ignoring Tylan. Of course, they were ticking the behaviour boxes, but nothing had really changed. Ty was a bag of nerves, frightened to go into school, never knowing when the next incident would occur. I wrote to the school again and pointed out their lack of meaningful work with these girls. I asked again for restorative justice work. It was then that an email went from the headteacher to the SENCo (Special Educational Needs Co-ordinator). It was sent to me in error, but I received it.

It said:

> Now stand well back and watch the fireworks . . .
>
> You do not have to reply to all of her emails, so when they come in, don't feel obliged to respond instantly until you have read and digested them or taken legal advice.[60]

This was devastating. But then, a lovely, nearly retired teacher in the school saw my email asking for help and responded brilliantly, putting together a piece of work with Tylan and the two girls who had bullied him. It was incredible. The girls cried and said sorry and made reparation. Ty was empowered and felt so much better as a result. The girls didn't bully Ty again. The whole activity took less than an hour and cost nothing. Using a non-violent resistance idea called 'The Announcement', Ty wrote down how he had enjoyed their friendship and appreciated their happy times in the past, but that things had turned sour. He explained how receiving their messages had made him feel, and then he ended with, 'This needs to stop and I would like to know what you or we are going to do to change this situation.' He read this to each girl individually, and by the time he finished, the girls were weeping. Each apologised and came up with a strategy to show Ty and other surrounding friends the difference they would make moving forwards. It was a beautiful piece of work. We will be for ever indebted to that teacher who was prepared to break the school rules.

Now, in 2017, we were renegotiating the EHCP with the school and we were seeing this 'take legal advice' attitude once again. We had managed to set up a situation where, if Ty was late getting to school, then a TA would sit in the missed classes, taking notes, then go through everything once Ty got there. A friend of mine had suggested we ask for something more. When Tylan couldn't make it into school for a few days in a row, the TA should come to the home and deliver the work in situ. I went for a meeting to discuss this. Around the negotiating table were the headteacher, the SENCo and the union rep, along with a man from the local authority whom I had never met before.

The school started the meeting with an absolute refusal to have the TA come to the home, threatening union action. I felt very afraid and intimidated, with no legal counsel. Little did I know that the guy from the local authority was a change-maker. He told them they would indeed be providing this service, and then he made them not only commit to it but organise a person on the spot and commit to letting me know when it would be arranged. He also told them they had a duty to write to me during the school holidays to let me know the latest updates. I could have hugged this guy. Everyone knows that if you have a SEND child, you are likely to get official letters about your child on the last day of the school year, leaving you to stew, unable to respond, for the whole of the summer holidays. This man had not only made them do their job properly but had also shown respect to me. All it takes is one person with the power to change things. It was a breakthrough moment.

All the same, 2017 was hard. There was also a lot going on for Nathan that year. He had been in the same primary school since nursery, and school had proved to be incredibly hard for him. He felt unsafe and on high alert. He would have violent outbursts, mainly aimed towards teachers but occasionally children. At the age of five, he had concussed his teacher, and when the school assigned him a TA, he broke the TA's fingers in a fit of rage. As a result of such high levels of violence, Nathan was not allowed into the classroom, and spent his whole day in the school gym. He preferred this arrangement because it was quieter, which meant he had lower arousal and could contain himself more easily. He feared his own behaviour.

All behaviour is communication. What was Nathan trying to tell the people around him? He couldn't read or write; he was really struggling academically and, like many adopted children, was way behind for his age. Adopted children have often had to spend a lot of their energy on survival and trying to get their heads around a cruel world. Sometimes, academic targets are not the goal for these children. Their challenging behaviours are inwardly screaming, 'Help me! I cannot tolerate this environment. I feel alone. Where are my family? Who are my family? Who can I trust? Why am I so different from the other children? Why am I so useless?'

If we can understand this could be happening, we can find compassion for the child who is deeply kind and caring but occasionally hits out. It was a very difficult time for the school and for us as a family, but the school tried hard to work with us to help Nathan. They were very compassionate.

One day, I was in the playground when a class mum came up to me and said, 'I'm so sorry about those parents with that WhatsApp group. I wanted you to know I never had anything to do with it.'

I was bewildered; I had no idea what she was talking about. Apparently, some of the parents had started a WhatsApp group in order to discuss Nathan. I then attended a school meeting with all the educational and adoption professionals present, and the headteacher spoke about 'the petition' she had received. Again, I was bewildered. No one had told me or David about this. Some of the class parents had signed a petition and brought it to the headteacher, asking for Nathan to be removed from the school. These were the same parents we chatted to every day. The same parents who shared their woes with us. The same parents whose children came over to play or attended our family events. People who we had welcomed into our space, who could very easily have spoken directly to us.

Nathan certainly had to leave the school – there was no doubt about that, he required a level of therapeutic care that the school wasn't equipped to offer – but this was not the way to do it. It caused real pain, and the sense of rejection was felt deeply by all of us. Sometime later, I met up with a group of adopters whose children had started in mainstream school and were now in special schools. They said, 'Oh, you had to do the walk of shame.'

I asked what that was, and they told me this was a common occurrence: you walk into school each day and you know people have had conversations behind your back; you notice people avoid eye contact so they don't have to say hello. This really resonated. We had walked that walk for far too long.

Like I said, there is no doubt in my mind that Nathan had to leave the school, but I felt sorry for him – and for his classmates, who really liked him. His friends had been taught to avoid him, to shun him, to reject him. What will we say of these children in a few years' time? These children who have been denied character-building experiences. We will accuse them of being snowflakes and lacking any resilience. Here was a chance, if only for a brief time, for them to show real kindness to someone different to themselves. A chance for them to understand some children really struggle with adoption. So often in life, we obsess over how someone metaphorically falls without considering where they tripped, or what they tripped over, or why. Too much of Nathan's life has been taken up with people judging his fall without considering where the issue started. He deserves compassion.

Of course, this school rejection did not help Nathan's self-esteem. He knew that people avoided him. This horrified him – and, more worryingly, it empowered him, in a sense. He had learned the effectiveness of fear, and that anger could be used to control other people's responses to him and as a way of avoiding acquiescing to their demands.

Working together with the professionals and the school, we found a place for Nathan in a pupil referral unit attached to a hospital. He would become a day pupil, travelling an hour each way every day. During the transition period, teachers would visit us at home.

So, by the autumn of 2017, we had three school-aged children at home with teachers visiting. Our home had become a school. Home-schooling was the last thing we would have chosen to do, because we didn't feel equipped, nor did we have the inclination. We have a number of friends who are super-gifted at it, but it takes a very special kind of person to do home-schooling well. The teachers would come for about an hour. Arlo would stay in their bedroom, so we would be left talking to the teacher. Tylan would be quietly learning with their TA, while Nathan would be running around hyperactively in the background with his new teacher. It was chaos! As people who had loved our own schooldays and were deeply committed to sending our children through the mainstream school system, it was a bewildering time.

Change in Crisis

On top of this, we now had two children who were experiencing suicidal ideation. Just trying to keep them alive, trying to access mental health help and make all the various meetings, was tough. When the aim of your parenting has become 'I just want my child to live', you know you are bumping along the bottom of life. When you notice your child who has no school to go to has carved the word 'stupid' into their leg, you know they are experiencing feelings of hopelessness. You must do something.

What could we do in this season of hardship? How could we get through all these challenges? How could we best serve our children and provide a stable, peaceful home? It was in this season that we dug even deeper inside ourselves. I remember crying out to God, 'Change this situation, change my circumstances. I cannot go on like this.' And then my prayer became, 'If you will not change my circumstances, then change me.'

And I changed. And we changed.

As full-time carers, we shape-shifted into therapists. We became teachers. We mentored, and restructured life, and found strategies, and worked hard every day to make a worthwhile life for our children. The delays in the system were the hardest part. Trying to access mental health services took ages, and then accessing any meaningful therapy took even longer. We found that health and education services don't really talk to one another, so there is no real collaborative leadership happening. In fact, we found, to our great dismay, that often we were actually the ones leading meetings; we were the ones asking the relevant questions and holding people to account, making sure that everything was done and that everyone understood the goals for each child.

The system is broken. School is often the place where the cracks start to appear. This is not to knock schools or teachers; we have experienced incredible examples of both. Some of the mental health workers we've met have been brilliant, and the local authorities can also do great work sometimes. But still, our children's lives are at risk as we wait for services to show up – and tragically, in our SEND community, some die in the waiting. When we look back and think about interventions and adjustments that could have been put in place when our children were younger, we see how different things could have been. If some money had been spent earlier, they would be avoiding the tens and hundreds of thousands of pounds of taxpayers' money services are costing now that our children are older and in dire need. Even if each professional does their job, children still fall through the gaps between services when there is a lack of any joined-up approach.

Having faced so much with our children, we have had to develop our parental resilience. Sometimes the events and new developments seem to be relentless, and adapting and learning while fighting to be heard can be utterly exhausting. It's important to remember we are also individuals who have needs. We can get lost in the fray. I often find myself very attached to my child's mood because I desperately want to understand them; it's as though I climb into their skin so I can work out what to do. While this helps my child, it's important that I remember to climb back out again. I am not my child, and I must continue to feed my own needs and re-establish my own autonomy. Sometimes, when I look at myself in the mirror, I look beyond the tiredness and worry and the rapid ageing I see there, and I remind myself I am still Carrie.

Similarly, many parents who are parenting together must remember we have our own joint relationship, the one we loved and nurtured before children. It's important to keep it alive in the midst of the mayhem. Sometimes (about three times a year), David and I will try to get away for a night, just to sleep and chat and eat without interruption. This is when we remind ourselves of who we are as a couple; we remember that we are in this together. With so many risks at home, it takes boldness to take this time out, and sometimes we must silence the accusing voices telling us we are bad parents for taking time to be together without children. I am also aware that some people may think this is a paltry amount of time to spend together – and you are right.

If we, as parents, cannot cope, our children suffer, so it's in everyone's interests to make sure we stay mentally and physically healthy. I yearn for a time when David and I have more space and time together, but in the meantime, we need to make sure our love still exists when that happens. Children, as wonderful as they are, can drive a wedge between a couple, so it's important to continue to feed the love we share and keep our vision of ourselves as a couple. To keep our 'us' strong.

First Responders

My writing has just been interrupted by Arlo sending a suicide message to me and David, and also to Olive and Tylan. Olive is away; Nathan is not in. Olive receives a message first and calls me. I run upstairs and Tylan is ahead of me, pushing open the bathroom door and snatching some antihistamine tablets from Arlo's grasp. We have four locked safes with medication in the home, and all razors and knives – anything dangerous – are locked away, too. Sometimes, it is incredible how children manage to lay their hands on these things. Arlo has taken two tablets.

Arlo is really struggling, and doesn't want me to tell them to live, that I love them and or that things will get better. They just want to shout and scream and express the big, uncontrollable, unbearable feelings. I'm just holding the space, nodding where necessary, from time to time repeating back exactly what they say, and agreeing with them that their life has been incredibly hard in places. David is calming Tylan, but Tylan wants to speak to Arlo. After about fifteen minutes, David brings Ty to the door. I'm not sure this is a good idea, but Ty looks determined and goes in.

Ty, at twenty years old, is incredible: empathetic, absolutely gets it, has lived through this himself, and says everything I couldn't say.

'You've not met the person who's going to be your best friend yet, Arlo. You've not seen the best scenery or even heard your favourite song yet.'

Somehow, these words are like healing balm and Arlo backs down, cries, and slowly recovers.

As I come back to writing, Arlo is now getting ready to go out to a local event with us.

That's how quickly these incidents can happen and turn around; it's business as usual.

For Arlo.

For me and David, it's chalked up as another incident where we have managed to intervene in time.

Was the threat real?

It doesn't matter whether it was real or not; people make mistakes in a moment they possibly won't get to live to regret.

My main concern now is for Ty, who must have been really triggered, and is off to Liverpool for work in the morning. I also let Olive know that everything is OK. Away from home, they must have been beside themselves with worry. As you can see, these things impact the whole family.

And what was at the root of the problem today? Eddie Munson, the character from *Stranger Things* to whom, as I mentioned earlier, Arlo really relates, was killed in the TV show. We had tried to stop Arlo from watching the programme; we had tried to find out what would happen with this character ahead of time, but alas, there were no spoilers. We tried to do everything in our power to avoid this situation, but somehow Arlo got to see that death scene. In their darkest moment, they said, 'I just watched myself die.' After today, they have agreed not to view this programme.

I do wonder how many other vulnerable children are affected by what they see and read. As a parent, you can try to protect your child, but there are always ways in which young people will do what they want to do; they will find a way. Arlo is quite rebellious. This comes from being out of school for three years. Now, the return to school has been like being a kid in a sweetshop. The world has changed in that three years – sex, drugs and rock 'n' roll! The friends they made online in the period they were out of school tend to be like them: the alternative kids who share and influence one another with their deepest, darkest thoughts.

What do we do? We have boundaries, times they must be home by (9pm). They must always keep their 'find my phone' function on. They always have a portable charger. We drop them off and pick them up from a lot of places. If they want to stay at a friend's, we make sure we have spoken to the parent. But you cannot monitor your child twenty-four hours a day. In one way, I am thrilled that Arlo has friends and somewhere to go, that Arlo feels they have found their people and can have fun.

We cannot control our children's every move, and there are always risks. It's about assessing those risks and having boundaries and a back-up plan. One thing's for sure: a vulnerable, edgy, cool sixteen-year-old will keep you on your toes.

What we are learning along the way

1. The human brain is elastic and new mindsets can be developed at any point.
2. Even the hardest of situations can be worked through.
3. Life is seasonal, and these hard times will pass. We can emerge at the end of a tough season wiser and more resilient.

Questions for the reader to consider

1. Are there areas in your life where you have grown in resilience?
2. Are there areas in your life where you want to become more resilient?
3. How do you use your life experiences to grow character?

7

FAILING

CARRIE

The real f-word in life is failure. The word we often fear the most; the word we do anything to run away from. If someone had asked us to write a book about how to be a success in the music industry, we would have very little to write. I have no idea how success has happened. We work hard, we keep believing, but apart from that, it seems to me that so much of our success has been as a result of taking the jobs that are a step down, or because the failure of one thing has led to the success of another. When we were singers for Take That, we would never have considered vocal coaching . . . until they asked. We felt slightly awkward about turning them down, as they were such lovely lads, so we went in with a high price, believing they would refuse, and then we could all carry on singing as normal. But they said yes – and the rest, as they say, is history.

Within a few years, we would be coaching numerous top

stars, we would have a best-selling vocal coaching book and a number-one DVD. None of it was planned. We just followed our noses and stuck with our desire to see artists cared for and performing at their best; it was all relational for us.

Last year, I presented at a big awards ceremony for a company with thousands of staff. One of the award categories was 'Biggest Failure'. I was confused. How could failure be rewarded? Then I saw what they were doing. Teams of people looked at an area of endeavour where the team had failed, and then assessed what they had learned from the experience, what they could take away and what they could avoid in the future. Suddenly, it made sense. Failing while facing forward, moving on and towards better outcomes.

No one wants to get parenting wrong. Feelings of parenting failure are common to almost every parent; we might feel that we have said something wrong, or taken a decision that wasn't right for our child. Often, parents feel as though they are not good enough, that they can't meet the needs of their children. Some people cannot manage being a parent for one reason or another, but all adoptive parents set out wanting to become super-parents. We all want to bring something solid and transformative to our children.

There are occasions when, in some families, a child's home setting is interrupted. We currently have a crisis in our adoption services. Adoption UK thinks as many as a quarter of all adoptive families are in crisis and in need of professional help to keep the family unit together,[61] with over 150 disrupted adoptions in each year.[62] There are no national statistics for failed adoptions, but it is estimated that the figures are between 3.4 and 9 per cent. Research by Adoption UK suggests about a third of adoptions encounter no significant problems, a third encounter problems but manage to resolve them, and the final third face challenges that are severe and ongoing. Another piece of research into teens shows that 30 per cent of adoptive parents experience regular adolescent-to-parent violence and abuse (APVA).[63] The most in-depth research into adoption breakdown, carried out by Bristol University, found that cases typically involved a significant degree of child-to-parent violence, running away and serious criminal behaviour.[64] In 2017, Department for Education figures showed that almost 15,000 families are using the Adoption Support Fund to help with crisis.[65]

So, what happens when parents face high levels of violence from their child? What happens when, as a prospective adopter, you attend adoption training, but no one tells you that you may face threats to your life, that you may be beaten up or threatened with a weapon? Two-thirds of adoptive parents experience violence or aggression from their child at some point.[66]

This is, of course, life-changing for anyone living in this situation, not just for the person who is beaten, but also for the rest of the family watching – and, of course, for the child. Everything I have told my children never to put up with, they watch me constantly put up with: allowing my son to beat me. As a parent, I am unable to strike back or push away; my only option is to curl into a ball and take the beating. We have been refused restraint training, so we have to manage the outbursts by risk-assessing them. The social services have intervened, but far from being the 'Team Around the Family' they are solely the 'Team Around the Child'. I have lost count of the number of times I have been told, 'Your child is at risk from harm because imagine if he seriously hurt you or killed you; he would feel bad for the rest of his life.'

The system is broken.

Nathan's early violence was difficult to manage at school, but at home we practised NVR, and it worked a treat. For five years, the violence left our home and was solely occurring in school. This is not to say the school couldn't manage; I think the school did somehow manage the violence. Nathan's challenging behaviour is not a daily occurrence, and most of the time he is delightful to be around. He hates school. He finds it hard to engage with learning – and, unfortunately, children who have violence as part of their profile tend to end up in schools with other violent children, so it's not the best atmosphere or setting for these children to be in. The issue for Nathan is that when there is an incident, it's on a big scale. There is something he feels in these critical moments that both terrifies him and empowers him. He feels omnipotent. The key challenge is therefore how to help Nathan to feel empowered and to understand his own agency without exploding.

There have been so many incidents in school over the years. Once, Nathan scaled the scaffolding of a neighbouring building and climbed to the top. All emergency services were called. The other children with him climbed down when things got a bit scary, but not Nathan. He stayed at the top for a full hour and a half, threatening to step off the scaffolding and into a burned-out shell of a house, putting his own life at risk. Afterwards, he would calm down and behave as though nothing had happened. There have been teachers who've had to spend their evenings in A&E, checking to see if their jaw, nose or some other part of them is broken. What can we do for this child? How can we reach him? We are super-trained up, the school staff are super-trained up, so what next?

Lockdown was very interesting to observe. School was online, we were all at home together, and our family thrived in this environment. There were no violent incidents for over six months. This is the longest Nathan has gone without an outburst, and there is something in this of which we need to take note. He absolutely loved being with just the close family, solely in one space, and with a relaxed but regular routine. Later in the year, he returned to school, and he hated it more than ever. On one occasion, he climbed on to the school roof and began to dislodge slates, throwing them at the school taxis waiting outside. On two occasions he absconded; we had police searching Hampstead Heath and helicopters overhead. It was incredibly stressful. Within a few months of lockdown ending, we were being called into school on a regular basis.

On one such occasion, when David and I had been called into school, Nathan became dysregulated at the school door. David and I were hit, punched, kicked and bitten, and I was eventually kicked in the face and knocked out. I had to go to hospital to have my face and head X-rayed. I had a concussion, but thankfully no cracks or breaks. But this act of violence towards me affected me deeply. As I lay there on the pavement, I knew something had changed in me. Perhaps it is different when professionals are injured. For me, it was devastating. I searched online for child-on-parent violence, but all the websites I could find were for adult relationship violence; there was nothing for this type of issue. All the support groups encouraged the woman to leave to get away from the violence. What was I to do when it was our child?

It's hard to explain child-on-parent violence or what it does to your mind. I have suffered a massive drop in confidence; I identify as a victim completely, and this is 100 per cent not how I want to feel. I survived my childhood and fought to make the transition from victim to survivor, but I never expected to be here again. So, this is the current challenge.

The violence we encountered in 2021 was the first violence we had seen towards us in years. In September 2021, we were told Nathan had to be permanently excluded, meaning he could no longer attend the school. He had caused £7,000 worth of damage to school property in one day. This P-Ex (Permanent Exclusion) was then changed into a 'Managed Move', meaning the school would be alongside him, providing education in the home rather than the school building, until a new placement was found.

A new placement proved hard to find, and within a few months, with no meaningful school experience, no therapy and no help, Nathan's violence returned to the home for the first time in five years. But this time, we were not facing a seven-year-old, we were facing a twelve-year-old, one who was bigger and stronger and with a harder punch. One day, he smashed up his room. It was completely obliterated: every cupboard door came off, every window blind was torn down, every breakable was broken, all the pictures were smashed. There was glass everywhere, and he was knee-deep in debris. David, Olive, Tylan and I just stood outside the room and waited for the emergency services to arrive.

The police arrived first. They entered his bedroom. He said he wouldn't come out; he threatened them. He hit and headbutted the police, and eventually had to be handcuffed. He was led downstairs and the ambulance service arrived. In fact, the whole close where we live was filled with emergency vehicles after they called for back-up. Twenty minutes after Nathan had calmed down, he went back to his room with the specialist paramedic, who was trying to assess how he was. Nathan looked at the carnage he had caused and said, 'Oh I'm glad my Pokémon cards are OK.'

The paramedics were concerned enough about his mental health to take him to hospital. He was put into a safe room, where he could continue to calm down and could be assessed. He then smashed open the mental health room door, and the whole of children's A&E had to be shut down.

Behind the scenes, David and I and the older children were desperate. We knew something had to change or someone might get killed.

We stayed at the hospital overnight. They brought Nathan a mattress and bedding, and I slept on the floor, with a security guard just outside the room. The next day, the psychiatrist asked for our family to have live-in security guards, but the social worker laughed at this idea, and rather than respond to the psychiatrist, said to me, 'Carrie, no one's going to swoop in to help you.'

So, no help came. Social services insisted that nothing could be done quickly. We would have to wait for them to write a report before they could help. A few weeks later, the psychiatrist diagnosed Nathan with disruptive mood dysregulation disorder (DMDD).

Symptoms include:[67]

- irritable or angry mood most of the day, nearly every day
- severe temper outbursts (verbal or behavioural) at an average of three or more times per week that are out

of keeping with the situation and the child's developmental level
- trouble functioning due to irritability in more than one place (e.g., home, school, with peers)

The previous summer, in June 2021, I'd applied to the Adoption Support Fund,[68] an organisation that helps a lot of families post-adoption. They were lovely and said they may be able to access some therapy for Nathan. They allocate up to £5,000 for adoptive families who need support. On applying, every therapeutic provider of the level we needed had shut their books because of being inundated post-Covid. As I've said before, in these situations, even if every person does their job, children may still fall through the cracks.

Two months and many violent incidents later, the social services report arrived. It was ridiculous. It was thirty pages long, and I sent it back with eleven pages of corrections. I was told no corrections could be made to reports. I insisted the changes be made, and asked for the leadership to speak with me. Eventually, most of the changes were made. In the report, all the emphasis was on me and David, and our ability – or lack thereof – to manage Nathan's challenging behaviour. Remember, we have been doing our expert work with no assistance, no school and no therapeutic input.

The school, on the other hand, were respected and affirmed for their strategy. Like us, they had a therapeutic approach, but they are professionals, so they receive respect and affirmation. Even if parents are also expert at what they do, this is never considered. As parents, everything you do is only ever seen as not enough. The school could restrain to protect themselves and others, but we could do nothing.

Our non-violent resistance training had helped us to manage the day-to-day, to de-escalate, and we used all the skills we had learned, but we had nothing for the major incidents. At this point, we risk-assessed the situation from a social services point of view. Having read the social services report, we knew how parents were viewed, so we made ourselves an assessment that could be written down, executed and reported. It was paltry.

- David would walk away from violence and move to another floor of the house.
- From there, David would call the police.
- I would take the blows from Nathan (the violence is aimed at me).
- I would curl into a ball to avoid my head being beaten.

In February 2022, that's exactly what happened. I was badly beaten up, taking multiple blows to my face, the back of my head and my body. The police asked why I didn't push Nathan away or defend myself, and all I could say was that I must 'think about the damage to the child'. I am not allowed to defend myself. The police were furious with social services, and told me that according to the law, I was permitted to defend myself. That was all well and good, but of no help to us, with a social worker looking at the damage to my body and still asking me to imagine how Nathan must feel.

At this point, Nathan was taken to hospital for mental health reasons. He didn't meet the criteria for a mental health unit, and he had no physical issues, so the hospital told us to take him home. We refused, and so we entered into a standoff with the hospital and social services. Social services told us our only option was to sign a Section 20 Agreement.[69] A Section 20 Agreement is where a child goes back into the care of the local authority, although the parents maintain ultimate control. At the time, I think this was probably a threat to make us feel like we had to take Nathan home. They had no idea how desperate we were. Nathan is and will always be our child; he is and will always be part of our family.

The idea was that Nathan would go to a therapeutic school all year round. We would visit him there, and once he could manage and get on top of the violence, the aim would be for us to begin to bring him home at weekends. This felt like an awful option, but our only option.

Three weeks later, on a Friday afternoon, without any notice, we were told Nathan was going to be moved. From Monday, he would live in Birmingham, in a residential home with no school. This was far from being a fifty-two-week therapeutic residential school. It was presented as a fait accompli. No collaboration with parents, no keeping us in the loop. At 5.55pm on a Friday night, we were told to sign the Section 20 Agreement immediately. We refused. We wanted to be given an opportunity to see the place and talk to the staff.

We spoke to the staff the next day, Saturday, two days before the proposed move. The house was for two occupants, one of whom was a seventeen-year-old boy. We asked why the previous child was leaving, and were told the child had become involved in a local county lines gang, so had to leave. This did nothing to assuage our fears or make us feel everything would be OK for Nathan. We decided to turn it down. The hospital and social services were furious with us.

This is what happens when people do not include the

family in their decisions. We spent another week in the hospital, waiting for some other form of help to emerge. Finally, it was decided that social services would provide two security staff in our home, seven days a week. The very thing the social worker had laughed at three months before.

We had security living with us during waking hours every day of the week. Two men from a pool of about six, in the house all day, every day. As you can imagine, this was not easy. The guys were lovely, but it's not normal to live with security, especially for our other children. Nathan would not engage with the guys at all. They were willing to take him out to do different activities, but Nathan did not want to engage. He became more withdrawn. His moods were dark; he was brooding all day, waiting for an explosion. He became more verbally threatening during this period, throwing things at me and threatening to kill me.

Simply restraining a child does not teach that child how to regulate their emotions. In fact, it sends the wrong message. It says, 'Don't worry, if you are violent, we will stop you, we will protect you from yourself.' It has no value in helping the child to work through his complicated and extreme feelings – and in the long term, when the 'restrainers' have gone, what then?

It was at about this time that David and I met up with a friend who had adopted several children and spoke specifically of one who'd had to return to care. He spoke of the violence from that child, and the way he and his wife had started to see changes in their own confidence and anxiety responses. I sat over dinner with a lump in my throat. I knew David and I could not go on the way we were.

Nathan deserves better. He deserves to have the support,

therapy and education that will help him to take his place in society and feel he has something to offer.

Our friend said, 'You guys have done incredibly well, and you look like you are coping. While you look like you are coping, the service doesn't consider you to be in crisis. You're not a priority. To access any help at this point, you will need to make it the social services' crisis.'

This made complete sense. We are not people who give up – ever. We just keep going.

As our public services operate in crisis mode, we don't really fit the bill.

But we were in crisis.

Total crisis.

Our other children were seeing this violence. I have been with David for over thirty-five years, living with a man who has never so much as called me a name, let alone raised a hand to me, and yet now I was facing the threat of violence daily. I could not go on.

The day after this dinner, a report landed in my inbox: the 'Domestic Homicide Review into the Death of "Sarah"/2016'.[70] The report relates to the death of 'Sarah' (aged forty-five), from the north-east of England, who was killed in November 2015 by her sixteen-year-old son 'Michael'. It was a very hard read, but it was important. We knew we had come to an impasse.

A few days after this, Nathan exploded, smashing our family computer. Thankfully, the security stepped in to stop him from getting to me. He bit the arm of the security guard, drawing blood, and threatened to kill me. Emergency services arrived. We ended up back in hospital.

The next day, we signed the Section 20 Agreement.

For twelve weeks, Nathan sat in the hospital, waiting for a placement. Now he really was the local authority's crisis. At weekly update meetings, we learned that the services were struggling to find a place that could meet Nathan's needs. We had to hear how the hospital staff were traumatised by watching Nathan in his room, waiting. Parents are expected to endure a lot. Not just to carry the weight of their own feelings but also the feelings of everyone else around them.

What feelings does this raise for him? Feelings that he is alone again and without family. That this is the end of the road for him. That life will now be a lot harder. He must feel abandoned, but we had no way back, and at this point there seemed to be no way forward. The social services thought they had found a place for him at one point. It was in Hull. There was nowhere near our home. In fact, there didn't appear to be anywhere within a two-hour radius. If he had ended up somewhere like Hull, a nine-hour round trip from London, how would we manage to see him? How would his siblings visit?

The system is broken.

The system does not support families to make these situations work. More money will be spent now than ever needed to be spent. I could take him to Harley Street for therapy every day and have private tutors all day long, and it would still cost less than the service he now requires. And Nathan, who is still a part of our family, still a 'Grant', is lost in the system.

There are no winners, only losers.

While Nathan sat in hospital, there were days I wanted to drive over there and pick him up. One week, I had Covid.

David didn't have it, so he slept in Nathan's bed. As he got in, he found a knife down the side of the bed. We have no sharp knives in our home, having locked them all away for our own safety, so I am unsure where this knife came from. But it reminded me that we had to keep moving forward with the decision we had made; we had to keep fighting to get Nathan the help he needed. We are so aware that once he is a little older, the violence will not be tolerated, and then he will potentially encounter another system: the criminal justice system. We want to avoid this at all costs.

For a period of time, we had to watch our son's life disintegrate. It was painful. Sometimes parenting is very painful. There is no doubt about that.

But there is always hope. Nathan is now in a therapeutic placement with a school onsite, set in beautiful countryside, with amazing staff. The home is wonderful, and they have not restrained a child for over nine months. This says a lot. They are clearly doing something that works. Looking at the placement, I can see why it's working: the mixture of staff, who are all very relatable, a good-sized house with very few items to smash, and surrounding fields that allow the children to get outside and think. The school is a forest school, which really works for Nathan. He picks berries and then makes a pie, gardens and helps the teachers. So far, Nathan is loving it. We visit him regularly. He is settled and back to being his sweet, affectionate and loving self. We have amazing times together as a family, wonderful walks in the countryside and long, uninterrupted conversations. The violence is still there in his current setting, but with a high number of therapeutically trained staff, Nathan is learning how to regulate his emotions. The physical setting makes it possible to learn and practise the tools he needs to get through life safely.

He is also engaging, in a meaningful way, with school for the first time. And the great part is that he is able to come home for overnight visits. Bit by bit, we will get him back into the home setting, first for weekends and then school holidays, at least. This is a necessary interruption to his story, but one that we hope and pray will work for good in his life. He will always be a Grant. He's our child, he's part of the family, and we adore and appreciate him.

When we feel we are failing, it is important not to lose hope. We hold on to the fact that when Tylan was ill, we couldn't imagine a future with him in it, and yet here he is now, largely thriving, working, living his dream. I look at Olive and I see the years of school criticism have been washed away, and now here stands the most incredible and wise human. And then there is Arlo.

Arlo, who had no school for three years.

When Arlo was first excluded from school, I visited an autism school in our local area. It was full of boys, and it was based in a house, which felt a bit cramped. Arlo did not want to go to the school. During lockdown, three years later, the headteacher texted me and told me about the new upper-school site and the cohort they had grown there over the past three years, which was diverse with regards to gender and sexuality. The headteacher told me there was one place in Arlo's year. She asked me if we would like to come and have a look. Arlo walked in, took one look, and said, 'I want to come here.'

Arlo, who would have a panic attack if the word 'school' was mentioned, was asking to go to this school.

In September 2020, Arlo went back to school. This school is amazing, understanding, patient, creative, quirky, and everything a teenage autistic child like Arlo needs. On day one, Arlo walked into the school. Everyone had masks on because of Covid, and Arlo marched up to the new upper-school headteacher and said, 'So, can I still come to this school if I get my nose pierced?'

It was a moment of testing, and I wondered how the headteacher would respond. A lot rested on whatever she was about to say.

She slowly pulled down her mask, revealing a nose piercing, and said, 'Well, if I have one, I don't see why you can't have one.'

I could have hugged her on the spot. What a great person she was, and is. The whole teaching staff have this approach, and it's perfect for Arlo.

We thought Arlo was educationally lost for ever, but there was a place for them in the world.

David and I often talk about these 'And suddenly . . .' moments.

They are real and they happen. Things can be so wrong, and life can be very difficult, and yet something often arises from nowhere, and suddenly things begin to shift. It's vital to keep holding on to hope, to stay 'in the game' until those moments arrive. And it's equally important to recognise these moments when they do come.

We longed for a moment such as this for Nathan. We have planted so much that is positive into him, and he has worked so hard to trust and attach. Finally, out of the blue, that therapeutic placement arrived: a home with a school attached, highly trained staff, a handful of other boys, and all within

100 minutes of his home. This was Nathan's longed-for 'And suddenly . . .' moment.

Failure may occur, but that does not have to be the end of the story. We always hold on to hope. Nathan has his whole life ahead of him, and things can change. He has so many beautiful qualities, and we really believe in the best outcome for him.

When parents feel a sense of failure, it can affect the way we parent. In times of real hardship, we have tried to help ourselves by looking at the work of child psychologists Dan Hughes and Jonathon Baylin,[71] and the theory of blocked care. Sometimes, the challenges we face with our children can impact our parent/carer brain at the deepest level. As parents, we operate several inner systems that enable us to fall in love with our children, to be attuned to them, to be able to interpret them and their motivations and drivers. These systems help us to think positively about the relationship between us and our children and the physical care of our children.

But what happens when these systems are challenged? The Child Psychology Service[72] website has an excellent explanation of the depth and breadth of the potential outcome but essentially it means that, as parents, we can come to the point where we feel defensive, burned out, are reactive and sensitive, are unable to think creatively about solutions to problems, and feel 'closed down' and isolated.

These feelings are valid. Being aware of what is occurring in our thinking can be the first and biggest step to recovering our positive feelings about the relationship. Respite is important; we need space and time to think. As parents, we owe it to our children to look after ourselves. Therapy, group support or simply having a non-judgemental friend as a sounding board can really help.

DAVID

It was William Ritter who said, 'Failure is not the opposite of success – it's a part of it.'[73] I'm the living proof that that's true, as the majority of what I've learned has been through failure. Our parenting strategies developed because of failure, and my willingness to learn was born of the fact that what I already knew wasn't working. My knowledge base wasn't deep enough to carry the weight of expectation that parenting placed upon me. Failure has been a catalyst for our growth as parents. As a parent of autistic children, I learned that what was a perfect action one day was completely unsuccessful the next. I learned that whenever I thought I'd found an answer to the question, they changed the question. Much of what I learned to begin with was by a process of elimination: I would do something, it would fail spectacularly, and I'd make a mental note not to do that thing again.

I never had a present father, but I assumed that one of the roles of a father was to make things better. I felt instinctively that a father was supposed to fix things.

When one child was on suicide watch, I couldn't fix it. I couldn't silence the words of the haters that were shouting in their head. I couldn't forget my own contribution to their despair. The number of times I had dropped them at the school gate, overriding their reluctance, believing that being armed with the knowledge of their father's love would be enough. It wasn't enough, and as I watched them devolving before my very eyes, I knew that I had failed them.

When one child was trying to make me aware of the traumatic experiences they had secretly lived through, of the harm people they had trusted had done to them, I didn't pick up on their hints and signs. They were trying to share a pain for which they didn't possess a vocabulary, but I didn't read the signs. I didn't hear them. I failed them.

When one child with no school, no peer group, no friends and seemingly no future asked me what the point of trying was, what the point of living was, I had no compelling answer. There existed no compelling answer, but I still felt like it was I who was failing them.

Sometimes failure is just a 'sense'. A sense of failure doesn't have to be attached to anything in particular; it's just a nagging feeling that we should be doing more, we could have done this or that differently, we could have done better. 'Did I do the wrong thing?' The constant, nagging question that doesn't always have an answer because, sometimes, there is no single right thing that would have helped.

Sometimes, at some very important times, I failed them.

And yet I'm grateful to failure.

Failure drove me to want to be a better father. It made me listen more and better understand the children I was parenting. I stopped giving answers to questions my children weren't asking, and instead committed myself to trying to understand their concerns.

Failure helped to build my character. At the points of failure, I began to accept how much I needed to know that I didn't yet know. Not every parenting strategy is going to work every time for everyone – it's not an exact science – but the more arrows you have in your quiver, the greater your chance of hitting the target.

Failure made me realise I had to let go of magical thinking. I couldn't hold myself responsible for the feelings of my children. I couldn't 'fix' the world for them. And, more importantly, if I failed to let go of the things I couldn't do, I would also fail to embrace the things I could do.

Failure made me more creative. If our children weren't responding to one thing, we had to come up with another. If one strategy wasn't connecting, we had to pivot and take a different direction. If a conversation was driving us down a negative road, we learned to head it off at the pass. Having strategies is one thing; having the creative instinct to apply them at the right time, and in the right way, is another, and it is often learned by trial and error. In other words, it's often learned through failure.

There is a saying: 'You never fail until you stop trying.'

Even the most successful parents have failed. Failures are not final if you learn from them. For us, our parenting failures and what we've learned from them have become essential stepping stones towards success.

CARRIE

We have never met parents more devoted to their children than SEND parents and carers. One thing they all talk about, especially when they first begin to speak up and share, are the feelings of overwhelming failure.

Often, this sense of failure comes from within, but it is also likely that it emanates from partners or other family members' judgements of them. Sometimes, it is from battling the school or services to get their child help; at other times, it may be that parents feel they are failing to be the parent their child needs.

'I don't like my child.'

From time to time, a parent will dare to utter these words. It is the boldest statement we hear. The admission that, in that moment or season, they are struggling so much they resent their child; they don't like the child they are raising. Often, these feelings seem to arise from being constantly verbally abused, or from watching other children in the family suffer because of the child who has additional needs or a disability.

We need to talk about this.

Parents are afraid of admitting to times when they regret parenthood, but there should be safe spaces in which parents can be brutally honest. Once the sentence is out, they can begin to shape it into a logical sequence, work out where things are going wrong and why they feel this way. In the safety of a support group, our darkest thoughts being heard can release a huge tension within us.

Not everyone has access to this kind of support, but Orna Donath's study *Regretting Motherhood*[74] is a good read, if only to hear from mothers who are reflecting on this tough issue. With this subject, there needs to be a space to simply sit with feelings without someone trying to 'bring you round' to being positive about your child. Again, as we often say, it is about our voices being heard, or just allowing the thoughts to come to the fore. There is a value in having a space where it's safe for suppressed thoughts to be articulated.

Raising a child with additional needs or a disability can be a challenge, and it is often within a community of like-minded, like-experienced people we find ourselves most comfortable. Extended family can be incredible, but in the experiences of people we've talked to, families often find it hard not to make judgements on your parenting. Granny may say, 'But they are wonderful when they are with me.'

This does not mean that Granny has the perfect formula; it just means that your child manages to mask for the time that they are with Granny, or that the change of environment helps them.

Then we come to the forgotten members of the family: the siblings. When a child has significant needs, all attention has to go to that child. Parents only have a finite amount of time and energy, and so often the child who demands less gets less. This child learns not to bother parents; they are natural protectors of their parents, and so make their own needs insignificant. They are like hidden carers, hoping that if they make no waves, everything will be OK.

Later, these children often have their own mental health crises. Sometimes, parents are late to notice because they, too, are relying on everyone around the child with needs keeping the status quo.

This is something we have had to apologise for with Olive. Being the oldest, Olive has a natural sense of leading and protecting. In Olive's late teens, when Tylan's life hung in the balance, Olive held in all their own needs. They felt responsible for Tylan at times, and fiercely protective over me and David. Olive could see what Ty's suicidal ideation was doing to us. Understandably, this sometimes led to feelings of resentment, especially as they had their own newly diagnosed ADHD to contend with. They were trying to come to terms with what this meant, they were trying new medications and they were struggling at drama school, and there was a whole lot of drama going on at home.

Children don't know how to take it in turns for parental attention – and nor should they – but when the family is in crisis, it's hard for parents not to become crisis-centred. The loudest voice gets the attention. Over the years, we have tried to make sure we are still listening to all the children, rejoicing with those who are experiencing breakthroughs while caring for another who may be in crisis.

In summary, failure is a part of being human, and therefore certainly a part of being a parent. Raising children is hard. Raising children who are different in any way is harder. Learning to move through failure is essential if we are to remain positive about our parenting. Placing too much emphasis on areas that are not a big deal, or over-focusing on things that we cannot change only leads to a negative mindset and is counterproductive. Knowing there are areas that may need change is realistic. Accepting we are doing our best in a situation that may be harder than we initially expected is still workable. Facing the fact that we are tired, mentally fatigued and out of sorts means accepting that we won't always knock it out of the park in our parenting. It's OK. Hope is round the corner, ready to meet us.

What we are learning along the way

1. It's OK to fail.
2. Failure doesn't have to have the last word.
3. We will all get through this.

Questions for the reader to consider

1. How do you respond to failure?
2. In what areas are you waiting for change?
3. What have you learned from failure that is usable in the future?

8

CONFLICT AND ANGER

CARRIE

We all have learned behaviours going right back into our childhoods that tell us how conflict should take place: the rules of war. One person may be an aggressive shouter, another may walk away from arguments with a door slam or a simple quiet exit, another may be passive aggressive during arguments, causing atmospheres that the whole family feel, creating their own hostile environment.

Conflict is hard, but it doesn't always have to be bad. Conflict can be good if it leads to resolution. Good conflict demands we experience uncomfortable feelings but commit to sitting in or working through those feelings until a solution is found.

The trouble most of us find with conflict is that it can quickly escalate and one or both parties 'lose it'. When we see our children escalating an argument, we make internal assessments about how we can turn the inevitable tide. For

Arlo, their teenage autistic meltdowns seem to be necessary to release built-up pressure. This means sometimes we will find ourselves in a conversation that rapidly declines into an argument where there is nothing being disagreed on; it's just that Arlo needs a safe space to vent. Of course, it would be an ideal situation if the pressure build-up could be released at a slower rate, thereby negating the need for meltdowns, but that is unlikely to happen all the time, and we have to accept that they will sometimes occur.

And what about our own anger as parents? What happens when *we* lose it? What does that look like? You'd have to be a saint for that not to happen occasionally. It's important to separate anger from acts of aggression. Physical interventions are not allowed in our home, but bit by bit, we have also eliminated aggression in the form of using intimidating physical presence. Standing over children or puffing up our chests: these things have gone too. Over time, we have also managed to get rid of raising our voices. Practising non-violent resistance really helped with this. First we de-escalate; we can then think through how we are going to deal with whatever we are facing in a calm way. The recapturing of parental control feels good, and gives a sense of reward. This means that 'losing it' no longer serves any benefit.

De-escalation

David and I have a 'de-escalation' mode. This is where we speak very quietly and very little. When we decrease our own volume, it means the shouting coming at us is met with deflation. It's very hard for someone to keep shouting for any length of time when there is a quiet, reasonable voice being returned. We then practise the communication model, repeating back what is being said or shouted. If a child is being totally unreasonable (and most of us are unreasonable when we've lost it) we simply quietly repeat what they are saying, however profane. This tells them we are hearing the words, and it also reflects how shocking those words are, especially if they include name-calling or judgement about us as parents.

We may also say something like, 'I can see you are upset. I'm sorry you are upset. If I have done anything to make you upset, I am sorry.'

Noticing the mood they are in and letting them know we notice helps. The word 'sorry' is like a balm, even in the midst of an argument; it prepares the way for later conversations.

There is no point in asking an angry person to tell you the true reason why they are upset if they aren't ready to share. If our children are in vent mode, they just need to let out the frustration. They haven't yet learned the sophisticated way of doing this. It's not reasonable, it's not measured. It's visceral and blurted. We have found it most helpful in these moments to 'hold the space'; to stay in the room and listen or leave if asked to. Anything to de-escalate. In these moments, this is the only goal.

We never try to teach our children a lesson at these emotionally charged times, nor do we try to give parent-to-child advice. They won't be able to hear it in this moment; that is for later, when things are calmer. Our children need to find a way to emotionally regulate. It's important to notice how they do this, and to recognise the signs for when they are struggling to regulate, both in the build-up and when we can see them trying to calm down. 'You're doing great,' can help in these moments, but it's really about finding how your child works at such times. Nathan needs to be left alone to calm down. Arlo needs us in the room, experiencing every bit of the vent until it passes. These moments can last anything from five minutes to an hour and a half, and sometimes we can feel them bubbling for days.

Strike While the Iron's Cold

This non-violent resistance (NVR) strategy is such a good one. In high-drama moments, we know that children cannot hear parental teaching, but this does not mean we ignore bad behaviour or abuse. In a way, there's no such thing as bad behaviour, just bad communication. When our children present with behaviours that challenge us, it's important to ask ourselves what they are trying to say. The behaviours our children present with can always tell us something. If a person has a communication problem, then it is likely they will present with behaviours that could be challenging.

Sometime after an explosive moment has occurred and been de-escalated, we will sit with our child and go over what happened, taking a moment to go over things once the heat has died down. This empowers parents and children alike.

We may have people on the sidelines of our lives shouting, 'You're letting that child get away with murder.' Perhaps if we were solely non-violent that would be the case, but *resistance* is an important part of the whole NVR way of doing things. What does resistance look like? Resistance is confronting the behaviour that we are working on or looking at situations where the child is out of control, and working out what happened and what needs to change. The heat of the moment is not the time for this, but afterwards, when our children are more capable of reflecting, there is an opportunity for us to speak.

With Arlo, I have said, 'There are certain swear words you use when you are angry with me that hurt me.'

If I said, 'There are certain swear words you use when you are angry with me that are really offensive,' this would have absolutely no impact on Arlo. They would automatically become defensive and accuse me of being easily offended. But Arlo understands hurt, and often when I have said this, they have managed to go a good few weeks without using the ultra-offensive swear words in the midst of a meltdown.

The main questions we ask post-explosion are: what happened here, and how can we do this better?

What Not Why?

As parents, it is so tempting to shout, 'Why did you do that?' or, 'What's wrong with you?'

The word 'why' in this context makes no sense to most children, but especially little to those who have had early childhood trauma. How can they possibly access those early years and answer in any coherent way? They are highly unlikely to be able to say, 'The reason I hit my teacher in school today was because when I was a baby . . .'

'Why' is too vague, whereas 'what' is concrete, allowing the child to tell the facts of what happened . . . not that they always remember these well! If a child is telling the story of events, they will probably describe the emotions they were feeling as a by-product of this sharing. They are more likely to be able to reflect on what went wrong and when, and what might need to change in the future for a better outcome, including their own responses.

The Sit-In

This can be a very helpful strategy post-conflict, especially when you are working to a target behaviour. When Nathan was six years old, he really needed to stop allowing his anger to boil over into violence, so we decided to perform a sit-in. This really pushes the resistance idea. We entered his bedroom. David said nothing; he was there to support me.

I said to Nathan, 'We've come in here to ask you to think about the hitting you have been doing. We want to work with you to find a solution, and we'd like you to come up with an idea that might help you to stop the hitting.'

The first thing he did was throw every toy he owned at me. I caught most of them, but stayed put. After he'd worn himself out, he then said, 'I'm going to fly to the moon.'

I told him this was not an idea that would work.

'I'm going to blow up the house.'

Again, I told him this was not a good idea, and that he had to come up with something better than that.

We all waited a bit longer, and then Nathan said, 'I'm going to walk to where the blue sofas are and lie down till I feel calm again.'

'Yes!' David and I cried. 'That is a great idea.'

From that day to this, we will often find Nathan 'calming down' on the blue sofas.

Working with our children and encouraging them to come

up with ideas teaches independence and shows them how to be solution-focused. It orientates them towards the right behaviours and responses.

Punishments and Rewards

There is much debate over the subject of punishments and rewards. Some parents swear by a star chart, others insist that all bad behaviours must be paid for, whether that's with the naughty step, no tech, no sweets or no treats. What we have found is that with our particularly wired children, especially Nathan, the concept of rewards and punishments creates high levels of anxiety. Worrying about getting something right, losing something, or trying desperately hard to win something just doesn't lead to better behavioural outcomes for our family.

What we do have are indiscriminate acts of kindness. Leaving a little box of Lego or Pokémon cards or a lip balm on a child's pillow so that they know we are thinking of them when they are out of the home. This is very important for children who struggle with outside activities, particularly school. We leave our children for six hours a day in the company of other children and adults who may not understand them, or at worst may be mean to them. To know that there is not a second of the day when they are not being held in mind helps them to get through.

To begin with, invariably, our children would find this little gift and would call out, 'What did I do?'

It's so interesting that they associated treats with good deeds, as if everything must be earned. While there is no doubt our children should understand the value of hard work leading to good results, there is a danger if we make behaviour our central theme, our children may feel like eternal failures: never quite hitting the mark, always under threat of parental withdrawal.

'I left it there because I was thinking of you and I love you. That's all.'

Most of us would agree that we want our children to know they are loved unconditionally, and unconditional love is modelled with this action. There is no performance required; they got it because they exist and because we love them.

We then began to get one child to leave something for another child, and it was incredible to watch how relationships were repaired by both the action of giving and the action of receiving.

Taking Responsibility: Blame Without Shame

DAVID

Show me a relationship where there's never been an argument, and I'll show you a relationship where at least one person has never fully expressed their opinion.

Although it's a fact that words give a semantic reality to thoughts and feelings, they can also limit our ability to fully express those thoughts and feelings. Even if we speak the same language, we may not share a mutual understanding of the meaning of words. A word that is neutral for one person might be so loaded with negative connotations for another that it triggers a reaction that, to the outside world, might appear to be bewildering and disproportionate. Easy and relaxed conversation can almost instantly become adversarial with the use of a triggering word or phrase.

Some people believe the spark that keeps their relationship exciting is ignited by combative communication, but that's not us. At the start of our relationship, Carrie and I connected on such a deep level, and with such mutual vulnerability, that the potential to devastate each other's lives was almost immediately present, and grew exponentially as our love and trust grew. The primary purpose of communication within a relationship is to know and be known; a potentially negative secondary aspect is that the more a person knows you, the more ammunition they have that can, if they wish, be used against you. The more aware they are of your weaknesses, the more precisely they can target the emotional weapons that you, in trust, have armed them with – and the more they can hurt you. If you've ever been hurt by someone close, someone you let into your secret world, the likelihood is you will be reluctant to reveal sensitive areas again.

When Carrie and I met, we approached the sharing aspect of communication from opposite perspectives. She was an open book and I had been totally closed. Carrie had spent a lot of her childhood desperate for people to know what was going on in her home. As a result, when I met her, she didn't keep her life a secret. She would confidently own every triumph and disaster, every situation and circumstance.

I was like Fort Knox by comparison. I'd spent my childhood desperate to hide my story. Everything was a secret. I had only ever told half a dozen people outside my family my middle name; no way was I sharing the events of my life.

But by the time we met, I was in a space where I was desperate to disclose, to bring the walls down and have a meaningful connection. Carrie and I had both seen enough conflict in relationships, experienced enough of people using each other's fragility to wound, or to score a point or win an argument, that neither of us wanted our relationship to follow that pattern.

We met as two strongly opinionated people, with two different life stories. We were similar in so many ways, but different in others. We knew there were going to be areas where we'd disagree, where our outlooks, and the conclusions our life experiences and backgrounds had led us to, were bound to be different. We also knew that for us to remain completely open to each other, we had to learn how to disagree in a manner that allowed our opinions to be conflicting without us personally being in conflict. We knew we would have to find ways to be able to challenge each other's statements without challenging each other's status in the relationship. We consciously set out to ensure that conflict, when it arose, was managed in such a way that it was never a 'deal-breaker'.

We worked towards creating a situation where we became intentional about trying to do conflict well, and we set about achieving this in several ways. We found out each other's triggers – words or phrases that were rooted in past pain – and made a commitment not to use them. We also acknowledged that certain ways of speaking – tone of voice, volume – or physical stance can be perceived as threatening, and we committed to try and eliminate those from our communication, along with swearing, name-calling and phrases like 'grow up' or 'don't be ridiculous'. We also learned the difference between storming out and taking time out.

We made a mutual commitment to avoid these types of

inflammatory phrases or behaviours. Looking back, I can see we were setting healthy boundaries and negotiating the rules of engagement, but at the time, it just happened naturally, because we both desired communication on a deeper level than we had ever experienced before, and we both wanted to feel safe. It takes incredible trust to communicate in this way, and it only works if both parties are totally committed to it.

The height of an argument, with all the tension and emotion involved, is never the time to get into the nuts and bolts of how to speak to one another, so we would talk about 'how' to argue during times when we weren't arguing. We discussed why we argue and when it's useful. We talked about the point at which the objective of understanding and being understood is best served by having a cooling-off period. We tried to recognise tipping points, the moment where the objective ceases to be about trying to express an opinion and becomes more about winning the argument. This was an important distinction, particularly for me. I loved a good argument; it was like verbal fencing. I had to learn that if my need-to-win attitude had caused emotional wounds, those emotional wounds would still bleed even when the conflict is over – and then who is the winner? There are no winners.

We made a commitment to tell each other the truth about our feelings, and to say what we really felt when it was right to do so and with an awareness of the impact our words could have. This became key to our communication. Another major key was to remind each other, even in the midst of conflict, that we love each other. Carrie first introduced this in the middle of a disagreement. I was making what seemed to me to be an indisputable point, absolutely convinced of my rightness, in full flow, voice rising, when Carrie quietly asked, 'But do you love me?'

It stopped me in my tracks. 'What?'

'You might be right, but do you love me?'

'Yes, yes I do.'

'That's good, I just needed to know that.'

It completely disarmed me, and made me realise what Carrie had already grasped, which is that our love was bigger than any point I was trying to make. Speaking the truth in love means that love is pre-eminent, and it became standard practice for us to reassure each other, even in the middle of difficult communication, that our love was bigger than whatever it was we were disagreeing about or trying to find common ground on. We also both learned the value of asking ourselves three questions – attributed to everyone from Socrates to Buddha – before opening our mouths to speak:

- Is it true?
- Is it kind?
- Is it necessary?

If the answer to all three questions is yes, then it was something we could say.

We learned to read and interpret one another. To notice when we might need space, or might need to just silently share a space; to recognise when we might need practical help, or just need the other person to see that we are struggling and offer encouragement. Being able to sit with someone in a problem is sometimes more important than finding a solution. With the right support, we often find our own solutions. This lesson we learned together of just being present, or 'holding the space', later proved to be invaluable with our children.

How we communicate echoes our relationship. The relationship that works for us is one where there is a natural, unforced ebb and flow, where we speak and listen to each other, and prioritise one another without ignoring our own needs. Again, trust is key. Rather than co-dependency, where one person finds definition and purpose in being the needy one, with all needs being met by their partner, who in turn gains identity from being the saviour of the needy one, we try to practise interdependency: giving and receiving as opposed to giving and taking. Receiving speaks of gratitude, accepting something given in love, often at a cost to the giver. Taking, on the other hand, suggests an expectation and an entitlement, grasping for something whether it's offered or not. We try to give, secure in the knowledge that when we are running on empty, the other partner will step in and trade places with us. It's never all one way; that just wouldn't work for us. In an environment of healthy communication and interdependency, the roles switch in keeping with each partner's needs and the ebb and flow of life.

When Carrie and I are not unified, it really impacts both of us. After almost four decades, we are completely blended with one another and instinctively sensitive to each other's moods. Generally, we sort out most potentially divisive issues in the moment, dealing with challenges to our accord in real time. We have found this prevents minor problems becoming major ones, and conflicts becoming crises. Some issues that create disunity can last a few days, during which we are both trying to 'get back to the centre' and may be hurting.

Every now and again, there may be an issue that will take

us longer to process and to find a resolution to, and it is these issues we find ourselves returning to time and again as we seek a harmonious way through. For us, unity doesn't mean uniformity. We don't go over and over an issue with rigid inflexibility until one of us concedes. Instead, when we are approaching the same issue from different directions, we try to understand the other person's viewpoint (even if we disagree with it), and then we attempt to find a third way, one that is mutually acceptable to both of us. This often means we both have to shift.

I used to begin every such conversation as if I was in a debate, a contest, in which I had to present an irresistible case in order to 'win'. I found I could be adversarial without being remotely emotional, treating each disagreement like verbal tennis. But because I was starting from the perspective that 'I know best', I found that my objective was always winning the argument rather than reaching any level of mutual understanding. Getting Carrie to agree that I was right took priority over finding an appropriate and consensual solution. I now begin from the position that Carrie knows something I don't. As such, I am open to having my opinions challenged and swayed by new information or a viewpoint that I hadn't considered. Carrie has the same attitude. We both see differences of opinion simply as each of us voicing what we consider to be best for the collective rather than jostling for primacy in the relationship.

Finding the Same Page

Parental unity doesn't just happen, it's forged over time – and in our case, was tempered and sharpened in the furnace of challenge. Like all new parents, we were completely out of our depth with our first child. Here was Olive, this unique, singular, stand-alone human for whom we were responsible, and somehow, we were supposed to just 'know' exactly what to do and when to do it. We were completely new to it, but we had a plan that we were determined to stick to. But of course, everybody has a plan – right up to the moment that it doesn't work, at which point they must devise an altogether different strategy.

When, as a first-time parent, you are in a sink-or-swim situation, learning to swim should give you confidence to carry into your next parenting experience, and so it proved. We parented our second child, Tylan, in a similar way, and, superficially at least, it seemed to work. We couldn't help but notice a few quirky differences to Olive, but not enough for us to realise that the way we were being read and understood by Tylan was completely different: that because of their neurological characteristics, their experience of us as parents was poles apart from the one we thought they were having.

What if your next parenting experience really is completely different? What if you are forced to learn a completely new method of parenting? Or what if one of you wants to learn a new way and the other one is unwilling?

This is the position in which we found ourselves. By the time we received the autism diagnoses for Tylan and Arlo, our parenting map was no longer fit for purpose, but I still clung to it. The raised voice, the flinty look, room time, the naughty step: none of it worked any more. Having recognised this, Carrie had moved on.

But I wouldn't; I couldn't. I was stuck, and we were divided.

Carrie and I had such a strong connection and an

instinctive understanding of one another's upbringings, and from the beginning, we'd had shared values. This extended to our views on parenting. We had always espoused the same worldview – until, suddenly, we didn't. From constantly being on the same page, we weren't even in the same library.

Carrie, with her mathematical, ordered brain, had audited, reviewed and analysed our parenting, and had identified several areas where we were clinging to practices and attitudes that weren't the right fit for our children. She was correct – we did need to evolve to meet the changing needs of our young family and our own understanding of the children we had – but I was overwhelmed by the new, unfamiliar parenting terrain we were entering. I didn't like the fact that, as a parent, I had to change. I wanted my children to change.

Being 'present' to me meant living in a world I hadn't signed up for, and a family where I felt disempowered, where I had to adapt. If this was the present, I didn't like it and I didn't want it. I wanted the days of 'yes' and 'no'; I didn't want 'perhaps,' and 'let's talk about this'. I wanted the past, when my word was law, no ifs, ands, buts, or maybes. The past was all the security I felt I had. I didn't want to move forward; I wanted everything to change back to what it had been. So, we did a metaphorical dance, with Carrie taking two steps forward and me taking two steps back. All the time, Carrie was trying to move into a parenting style that suited our children's needs, and I was trying to hold on to a parenting style that suited my upbringing.

When I was growing up, nobody had asked my opinion; why should I ask my children theirs? Back in the day, if a child shouted at their parents, every black adult would say,

'Why do white people let their children shout at them?' I wanted to be the cuddly but slightly scary dad to whom kids wouldn't dream of being rude. But that ship had sailed, and although it was clear my old way wasn't working, I honestly didn't know what would.

Carrie and I had come to an impasse, and because of our lack of a cohesive parenting vision, the message the children received would depend on which parent they were speaking to. When decisions needed to be taken quickly, we would sometimes even heatedly debate whose parenting strategy was correct – right in front of them. Yep, we did that.

I've spoken to many co-parents who've felt at various times that their partner and children were on one side, and they were on the other. The feeling of things moving on and one parent being left behind is a common one. If Carrie and the children were all on one side and I was on the other, perhaps it was me that was on the wrong side; perhaps it was me that needed to change. I found it hard to shift, especially when, on my side, I had a large portion of logical society telling me my way was right. I clung so tightly to the belief that I would be a great dad to a neurotypical child.

I had access to countless books full of great parenting advice, libraries full of strategies, but none of the advice made a difference to my children or the success of my parenting. Put simply, when parenting neurotypical children, parenting principles, objectives and philosophies can be reassuring and give us a foundation and framework, but when we are living with children who don't fall within a typical neurological profile, what then? These 'different' children may require not one way of doing things, but several. What worked yesterday may not be working today, so our strategy for each child must be both made-to-measure and flexible. We have to be prepared to adjust our parenting style at the drop of a hat.

Neurotypical children flourish with consistency. Neurodivergent children may also want that consistent element, they are often very reliant on routines, but how that plays out in practice may also change at the drop of a hat. For instance, Arlo likes to have a thirty-minute drive every evening, this provides a kind of scaffold for their mental health. Some days Arlo may decide they want it at 6pm and others at 10pm. Some days for no apparent reason, ten minutes into the drive, they insist on returning home immediately. On another day, for no apparent reason it has to be a long drive. There are no patterns or events during the course of the day that can prepare us for these changes in routine but when they happen we have to respond to them as there is no telling how much of Arlo's immediate emotional stability is invested in these small but unexpected changes. We have to be both consistent and flexible and also prepared for the day when Arlo says they no longer want a drive, they want to go to the gym every evening. I have had to adjust my thinking and accept that the parenting style I was practising was perfect for neurotypical children – but I didn't have any neurotypical children, so it just wasn't working. The challenge now was to start parenting the children I had, not the non-existent ones for whom I had prepared.

I was going to have to revise the whole metric by which I measured good parenting and reverse the philosophy that demanded my children conform to my pre-set definition of correct outcomes. I had to find out who they were, not just who I wanted them to be.

Reluctantly, I had to begin the long but necessary journey.

If I was going to lead our family alongside Carrie, I had to be prepared to humble myself enough to change.

I couldn't hold back the tide. This is where NVR, something that we could work on together, came to our aid. Mending broken communication took desire, effort and time. Sometimes unity is hard won, but if you are in a co-parenting situation, it's essential, so it's worth fighting for.

Forgiveness

For many people, 'sorry' really does seem to be the hardest word. It's seen as a capitulation, an admission of defeat, a climb-down. In viewing the word so negatively, people fail to appreciate its healing power. 'Sorry' is not an indication of weakness, it's a soothing balm. 'Sorry', spoken sincerely, is an invitation to reconciliation. It's an indication that our shared humanity means that none of us is right all the time, and that when we are not, we have the courage to admit it.

The power of a sincere apology is one of the greatest gifts my mother gave to me. If she discovered she was wrong, she would say so. It meant that I never doubted her integrity, and that I saw her as strong because she was never afraid to admit her fallibility. If she held firmly to an opinion, it was because she really believed she was right, not because she needed to win. She owned both her strengths and her weaknesses, and that is something I have tried to replicate, both as a husband and as a parent. The power of 'sorry' has become a natural part of our family discourse. We can all – adults and children – withdraw an erroneous statement or wrong action without having to climb down, without feeling shame and without being exposed to ridicule.

The other side of the apology is the response, because apology and forgiveness go hand in hand. If sorry is the hardest word, to forgive is, for many, the hardest action. I know this from first-hand experience. I spent years harbouring the resentment I felt towards my father, nurturing my sense of abandonment and drawing strength from it. In moments when I felt like giving up, I would harness the pain of rejection to motivate myself. I felt as though I was using my hurt, cultivating unforgiveness and channelling controlled anger. I found out that unforgiveness comes at a cost; I wasted what should have been the joy of seasons of success in fearing failure. I was motivated by a need to prove that 'they' were wrong – but what if 'they' were right? 'They' were not just my father; the list had grown until it included anyone who, at any time, had expressed any doubt in my ability to succeed. The thing is, 'they' didn't have a clue that their doubts were fuelling my drive away from failure and penury. I attempted to use unforgiveness as a catalyst in my success. The drawback to doing so was that I had to stay angry to stay motivated. It was emotionally exhausting. I was replaying unkind words, criticisms and hurtful moments on a loop in my head, just to push myself to never go back there, to never be in a vulnerable position again. Unforgiveness does that: it traps us in the prison of the past and throws away the key.

Forgiving nothing makes us a shell of the people we could be; it destroys us psychologically. If we are clinging to the past, we will never be free to embrace the present. It's only by being in the present moment that we can create our future – and if we are holding on to the past, we can never fully be in the present. Occasionally, when I was growing up, my mum would refer to her past hurts. Words, situations and events that had damaged her. It's hard for children not to imbibe and be influenced by the big concerns of their primary adults. My mother's fears became mine; her financial fears made me afraid of being without money. Her feelings of having to fight for respect as a black, single mother in the London of the 1960s and 1970s made me sensitive to slights both real and imagined.

There were so many things my mum rightly refused to accept, and I inherited her acute recognition of injustice. But I also inherited her anger, triggered by her experiences, and I would carry it into the next generation, along with other baggage, such as a fear of rejection and a resignation to ultimate failure. My mum's unwillingness to let go of the past meant that the outcome of each new experience was filtered through past experiences, rather than seen as a fresh, stand-alone event. When I was about to become a parent, I knew that I couldn't pass my inherited unforgiveness issues on to my children. Forgiving the past or remaining enslaved to it became my only options.

I learned that forgiveness sets us free from holding on to pain. The more we love and the more open we are, the more susceptible we are to being hurt. Raising children together requires unity. Trust is an essential part of unity, and trust and forgiveness go hand in hand. Because of the vulnerability love creates, our partners and our children may sometimes behave in triggering ways, causing anger or uncomfortable responses in us. It's important to remember that even though they have accidentally – or deliberately – pushed the buttons, they didn't *create* the buttons that have been pushed.

It is always harder to forgive when the person who needs forgiveness shows no recognition of wrongdoing and expresses no remorse. It's important to remember that forgiveness is not acceptance. Forgiving doesn't condone or let the other person off. In fact, forgiveness has very little to do with the other person. What was wrong may still be wrong; forgiveness is what we do to release ourselves from being held captive and shaped by the wrong that was done to us. Forgiveness is the first step in breaking free from the captivity of pain.

Forgiving ourselves is essential. In fact, until we can forgive ourselves, it makes it difficult to forgive others. Forgiving ourselves is a part of recognising we are not who we were. We can forgive the choices we made yesterday because we are different people, who would make different choices today. Wisdom doesn't prevent us from making mistakes; on the contrary, wisdom grows as a by-product of making mistakes and learning from them, forgiving ourselves for them and moving on armed with the wisdom that comes from having made them.

The parent you are is an extension of the person you are. An absence of self-forgiveness leaves us holding on to the person we were. To become the best parent we can be today, we must forgive and let go of the worst of who we were yesterday.

Forgiveness frees us from being tied to the painful past. Sometimes, the best and safest decision for our children's sake is to walk away from a relationship. Learning to really understand our different children and then becoming a bridge between them and a world that struggles to understand them is made harder when one partner doesn't want to understand, or is more committed to changing the children than to discovering them. There are as many reasons why relationships fail as there are failed relationships, but whatever the reasons, moving forwards into the new, starting again and rebuilding are doubly difficult without forgiveness. Without it, we are still holding on to what we've left behind – and it's still holding on to us. Past bitterness cannot be the foundation for future joy.

What we are learning along the way

1. We can all improve the ways in which we communicate, especially during conflict.
2. The goal is not to win but to understand one another.

Questions for the reader to consider

1. How do you respond during conflict, and what do you hear that may not be there?
2. How easy/difficult do you find it to forgive?
3. How easy/difficult do you find it to say sorry?

9

Purpose and Hope

CARRIE

Love and relationships are often what drive our lives, but purpose is also super-important. There is day-to-day purpose: what we are all up to, being busy, doing this and that, holding down a job, having friends, family, relationships. And then there is deep purpose: what we will call sacred purpose. That part of you that comes alive when you are doing what you were always meant to do. Hitting the sweet spot in life and knowing this is what you are here for. We cannot talk about parenting without talking about purpose. Introducing our children to the concept of purpose builds that part within them where love and community can effect change. Our children can be world-changers if they change even the tiniest thing around them. Caring for our world and those who live in it is a fundamental part of purpose. Purpose can lead to us feeling a deep sense of satisfaction that isn't based in the normal drivers of status, money and recognition. Caring about the legacy we leave is very important to me and David.

As parents, we teach our children to regularly think about purpose. What's the thing that you do best out of all the things you are interested in? Is it connected to people, creativity, community, faith or a particular gift or skill you possess? Finding your purpose changes the world. That is not to say we are all going to get out into the world and be 'famous for it'; it is about getting to a place where we feel we are flowing and our gifts and skills make sense and have context. On a more earthly level, my parents would have said having an interest kept us kids out of trouble, and I think to a certain extent that is probably true. We were too busy to be messing around.

I have always loved the arts. I am a total creative, the way I see the world is creative, but I know my real purpose – my sacred purpose – is to do with people and advocacy. I have found my own voice by raising it for my children, and in doing so have realised I can raise it for others too. This gives me great pleasure, and in the hardest times with the children, I know the suffering is crafting a better me – one who will speak up. That 'speaking up' may simply involve having conversations with others who are at the start of their adult life or parenting journey, or it may involve training leaders. Everything we have gone through is usable; not one thing is wasted.

Some of us know at a young age exactly what we want to do with our lives, others evolve our purpose, and still others find a driving force later in life. The latter was true for my father. I love telling this story, because my father's life evolved against the odds, against age, and against skill and knowledge, or even confidence.

My father left when I was seven years old. He ran off with Claire (name changed) on our family holiday at the Pontin's holiday camp. Like many children of divorced parents, at the time, I would see my dad every other weekend. In my teens, this went down to about once a month, and by the time I was in my early twenties, a few times a year. In 1988, I was twenty-two years old and knew I was ready to get married to my soulmate, David. I knew I would have to share this news with my dad. We sat down for dinner.

'Dad, I have something to tell you. I've become a Christian, and I'm getting married.'

The conversation developed; details were shared. My dad, who had no faith and was very narrow-minded, said, 'Well, darling, there are two things you need to know about me. I hate Christians and I hate black people.'

This was not going well.

David and I discussed what to do about my dad. The wedding was coming up, and we didn't want his negativity to permeate our joy. After a lot of consideration, we both felt that our love was bigger than any one person's attitude. We decided to be the bigger people and invited him. We had no idea, but extending a hand of grace to him in this moment would come to mean a whole new story emerging when, just two months after our wedding, devastation hit.

My dad had no one to turn to. He had never cultivated friends, never felt the need to confide in anyone or make a community. His entire life had been about being a husband (sadly, not a very good one), being stock-controller at the factory, playing golf on a Saturday and washing the car on a Sunday. He didn't make friends and didn't really even stay in touch with his wider family. He was an under-confident man who maintained any sense of worth by keeping his life as small as possible. He'd had a very difficult childhood with an alcoholic father. He was in and out of the Barnardo's children's home in Enfield as my nan tried to get her life together. As the only boy and the eldest in the family, he'd had to be tough, resilient and protective. And so he kept his life small.

'I don't know what to do. Claire has left me.'

This would be the opening sentence to the beginning of an incredible relationship between me, my dad and David. My dad was at a complete loss, with no sense of how his life could function without Claire. He had assumed he could neglect her and be rude to her, and that she would always put up with it and be there for him. He was wrong. He got up the next morning and made it into work. He had been in regular employment since the age of fourteen and had worked his way up. The action of getting out of the house was important at the time, and gave his life routine. Most nights after work, he would find himself at ours, having dinner. For the first time, I saw him cry. He would cry at how hard his life was, and weep at the kindness we showed him – especially David's kindness. My father was humbled by David's love and concern. We began to see a seismic shift in him.

Six weeks later, after a lovely Christmas together, my father asked if he could come to church with us for the New Year. This would be a big test, not least because many of the members of our congregation were black.

I sat in church between David and my dad and tried to work out what he must be thinking of all of this. He looked intrigued. A young woman got up to sing.

'Amazing Grace'.

Her voice was beautiful, ringing throughout the church, touching the hearts of the congregation with her passion. I slowly leaned back in my seat to get a side view of my dad and work out what he was thinking.

Silent tears rolled down his cheeks. He made no effort to hide them or wipe them away. He couldn't move. I had no idea what to say. I was at a loss, so I stayed silent and didn't interfere with what was happening. But something was happening.

After the service, my father told me that when he had been young, he had attended church. At the time, it was the only calm in a life of storm. He'd met a lovely girl and they had fallen in love, but then she left him to become a missionary. It had broken his heart and he vowed never to go back to church. He was angry with God. He met and married my mum on the rebound.

But here he was, nearly forty years later, with his heart uncovered and his soul calling out for relationship, for love, for something more than this life and all it had led to.

My dad started to come to church with us each week and made friends with our friends. He became a part of our community, and he absolutely loved it. It was as though all his social anxiety, all his lack of trust, had been swallowed up. He had found his people. His people were diverse and creative, young, vibrant and alternative. He loved them all and lavished friendship on each of them, building strong relationships outside of the friendships David and I had with them.

It was now 1989. In May of that year, my father returned to our home for dinner with another terrible announcement.

'I've been made redundant.'

I knew this was huge. My dad needed his work; he had always worked. He was fifty-six years old. What on earth would he do now?

But he didn't seem bothered in the slightest. It turns out, this was the push he had needed. He went on to announce, 'It's fine, because in September I am starting Bible college.'

Studying theology when he'd left school at fourteen years of age seemed like a mad idea to me and David. But off he went. And he thrived. My dad was finally using the brain he was born with. He was intelligent and loved studying.

Privately, David and I were wondering where on earth this study would lead. At fifty-eight years of age, my father would graduate from college – and then what?

Dad sat us down.

'I want to be a missionary.'

This was an insane idea! My dad ... a missionary? My dad, who could barely talk to more than two people at a time. Could he really go somewhere to talk to many people? He was a working-class Londoner, a lad, a cheeky chappie – without any cheeky.

'OK, Dad. So where do you intend on doing this missionary thing?'

David and I held our breath in anticipation.

'Sierra Leone.'

At this, David doubled over laughing. 'So, God takes a Christian-hating racist and makes him a missionary in Sierra Leone. What a great sense of humour he has!'

Even my dad could see the funny side.

Towards the end of 1991, at the age of fifty-nine, my father left for West Africa. He was no preacher, but he had loved his Bible college course, so he decided teaching would be the best thing for him to do. He was resourceful. He made friends with the KLM (Dutch airline) office in Freetown, the capital, and there they allowed him to photocopy his theology course notes for free.

He opened twelve Bible colleges in Sierra Leone.

Many of the missionaries in Sierra Leone live on compounds, drive four-by-fours and are well funded by their home churches and charities. Not my dad. He lived locally, ate locally and became known as 'the white man who walks'. He was loved and accepted. He had found his sacred purpose, and in doing so, had found himself.

It is 1996 when the police come to my door in London. They tell me of my father's death in Sierra Leone. He has died very suddenly of cerebral malaria. I am given the option to have his body flown back to the UK, or to go out to West Africa and bury him where he is. There is a civil war going on in Sierra Leone, but I decide this is the place where he belongs; this is where he shall be buried.

I take a flight, and as I sit there on the plane, I wonder what I will be walking into at the other end. I am met by friends of my father. I stay in Sierra Leone for five days.

It is hard to measure the impact my dad has had on people. There are literally hundreds of people at his funeral. In conversation, I hear the same phrases, over and over again.

'Thank you for lending us your father.'

'Your father was like a father to me.'

'Your father was a wonderful father.'

It is here, in this place, that I realise that everything he wasn't really able to be as a younger man, he has become in this last chapter of his life.

He went out triumphant, a winner, a giant. I truly love my dad for the legacy he has left me.

After Claire left him, he could have shrunk his life. He would have been justified in giving up. But in this difficult time, he faced his own inner giants, reached into his future and found a wonderful adventure.

It is never too late.

No matter how old we are, no matter how many challenges we have, there is always more to be had from life.

In 2008, David and I return to Sierra Leone with Comic Relief. We are in a café, and I am talking about my dad when a lady at a neighbouring table leans across and asks, 'Are you talking about Bob Gray?'

I nod yes.

And she tells me that some of my father's colleges are still running. Twelve years after his death, his legacy lives on. This is sacred purpose at its very best.

It's also never too late to change the narrative about yourself as a parent. Many of us feel we have failed; we have lost, or we just can't match up to demands. Yes, you can. You can do it. You can grow and change and evolve and become all you need to be. Sometimes, our desires are strong but our will to change remains static. There is always a moment when our desires and our will line up. We need to jump on this moment and grab it for all it's worth, letting it catapult us into a better place.

Hold on to hope.

It is one of the most precious things in life. We have fought to find the positive, and we've faced our fears. We have stepped into the unknown and travailed to reach a point of hope.

People speak of hope as if it is this delicate, ephemeral thing made of whispers and spider's webs. It's not. Hope has dirt on her face, blood on her knuckles, the grit of the cobblestones in her hair, and just spat out a tooth as she rises for another go.[75]

Some days are like this.

Some seasons are like this.

We have worked hard at embodying hope and fostering an attitude of expectation in our day-to-day lives. Sometimes, it's impossible – and that's OK. We all need time to sit down at the side of the track and rest. But, like I said, there comes a moment when we know we have an opportunity to lift ourselves up. It's about grabbing those moments.

And for those who are discouraged: things can change. There is hope. If you are that parent who feels like giving up, please don't. Remember, Arlo went from having no school to having a great school. Nathan went from having no school or therapy, or any proper outside help, to having a space that is really working for him. Olive went from struggling in a drama school where they were largely overlooked to working at the highest levels of our industry. Tylan went from suicide watch with no one understanding him to being a voice for many autistic people and an award-nominated actor.

There is a community of people out there who are just like you. You may not know them yet, but they are there. They are probably worrying about many of the same things as you are right now. They may be wondering how they can fix things for their child, or how they can be a better parent, or how they can grow confidence in their parenting. The world needs you and your family.

We sometimes wonder what our legacy as a family will be. We hope we will be an example of what a family looks like when people can grow into who they are created to be: an authentic, real-life, messy but beautiful family.

With small and simple acts of kindness, we hope our family can move among people whose lives are enriched for having walked some life miles alongside us.

One of the greatest areas of life for us is building community with others. We feel that building, joining or being a part of a community is essential to life. There are people who like to lead a solitary life, but even these people will often belong to online groups. Being able to see ourselves reflected in others is helpful; it makes us feel seen and heard. There must be places where we can show up as ourselves, where we know we are loved and accepted just as we are. Being a part of a group can make us feel purposeful, and lots more can be achieved when a group of people get together to effect change. We learn from one another when we face difficult times; we know we are not alone in our suffering. And when a group of people decide that change is needed and there are issues to be addressed, they can create a groundswell that acts as a lobby for transformation.

Ten years ago, we were asked by our local autism service if we would start a little group, once a month, for local families who had autistic daughters. There weren't many diagnosed girls, so for the first three to four years there were between ten and twenty people attending. Then things began to change as more and more females were managing to get assessments, and the group grew. We currently have about 180 families, and it is both a rich resource and a place where people can be their honest selves. The group comprises two groups: one for the parents (and grandparents or friends who are involved in the child's life), and one for the girls themselves. This latter group has also extended to trans and non-binary children in order to reflect what is happening in our community.

This group is like another family to us. The people we walk alongside bring hope and purpose into our lives. They have walked with us through some tough terrain, without judgement. They have been our cheerleaders.

DAVID

When it comes to hope and purpose, it's important to remember why we do what we do.

We are all either 'to' people or 'from' people.

'To' people are driven by the desire to move towards a destination. They are inspired by and curious about what lies ahead. They live in the present, and their energies are spent on dealing with the now and anticipating what's next. Their focus is primarily on always moving forwards, because they are excited by what's ahead of them. They are not driven by fear or pain about what lies behind them; they are driven by the hope and expectation of tomorrow. They are not focused on where they've been, but on where they are going.

'From' people are driven by the desire to move away from past events, feelings or circumstances. They are not primarily motivated by the thought of going towards what lies ahead, but are more driven by the desire to put distance between the present day and the past. They desire to get away from something, and they have a pressing need to ensure their future doesn't mirror their past. Their focus is primarily on never going back to the place they are moving away from.

Both sets of drivers can be powerfully motivating. The constant quest for whatever is next, the constant need to escape the past. Only one of these comes without fear. If you are a 'from' person, every mistake can feel like a rerun of past mistakes; every slip, trip or misstep can be taken as a portent of impending doom and inevitable failure. As a parent, this can be debilitating. The constant fear that you are not enough, don't know enough, that you're not wise enough, is inhibiting and self-defeating. The fear of reliving the past, with its deprivations and disappointments, can rob you of the joy of parenting and the joy of being alive.

None of us begin our parenting journey fully formed. Each child is different, so whether you are on your first child or your tenth, the journey will be unique. The principles may be the same, but the character, personality and identity of each child is different. It's these differences that make every parenting journey not just a voyage of discovery, but also a singular learning experience.

Each journey will require us to be a different parent, and by meeting these different requirements, we discover things within ourselves that we would otherwise have never known were there. Reserves of resolve, the capacity to press on in the face of sleeplessness, in the face of exhaustion, when we're running on an empty tank, but we keep going. The points where physically, we are spent, but we keep moving forwards on willpower alone. The moments when those to whom we look for encouragement don't understand us, our children or our parenting, but we soldier on because there is no other choice. Seldom do we ever realise that in doing what we are doing, in simply getting on with life, we ourselves are being changed.

Sometimes, I hear people say, 'I'm just a mum,' or, 'I'm just a dad, nothing special.' Yet what we are doing couldn't be more special. In the routine, in the mundanity, in the repetition of a parenting journey, we change, we evolve, we grow – and while doing so, we give matter to a child's dreams, we shape a child's destiny, and we build belief, even through the times when we have none ourselves. And in doing so, we change the world.

Some parenting journeys are hard, and some seasons are hard. There will be times when it feels like every time you find an answer, they change the question. We only grow through what we go through, and with each storm we have navigated, we have grown. Never underestimate the power of hope, and never undervalue the power of purpose.

Hope is essential for us as people and as parents. Although we put our children at the centre of our lives, it's important that we have hopes *for* them, but that our hope isn't *in* them. We know of parents whose lives have become so consumed in their child(ren) that they forget they are separate entities with their own hopes and purpose.

Purpose is at the centre of parenting. We might hope that a particular action works, that this strategy is successful and that each change we make is the right one, yet at the same time, our purpose – to be more confident parents, to be able to identify what works for each child, to exercise self-care – is paramount.

Purpose is at the centre of life. Each of us has a sacred purpose. It is the thing that aligns with our passions, gifts and talents. In life, each of us plays several roles – friend, colleague, partner, wife, husband, parent, sister, brother – and the function of each of these roles changes as time goes by. Our purpose goes beyond function. For some people, parenting is the pause button to purpose, the barrier to fulfilment of purpose, yet if we can bring the energies, presence and focus that we apply to our purpose into our parenting, it can change the parenting experience from one that is functional to one through which we can fully express who we are. Purpose and hope go hand in hand. If hope is our guiding light, then purpose is our compass. If we can build both into our parenting, then rather than being something to be endured, parenting can become the journey of a lifetime – storms and all.

CARRIE AND DAVID

And one final point from us, right back to where we began:

Be a rule-breaker.

Break the rules for the better. Change only happens when someone steps outside of the *normal* way. Be the person who says, 'We don't normally do this, but . . .' and change a person's life in the process. Keep thinking outside the box. There is no end to our creativity when we begin to imagine a better future for our family and the world.

What we are learning along the way

1. Our sacred purpose can arrive at any point in our life; it's never too late to discover yours.
2. Purpose can get us through some of the hardest times and situations we face.
3. Sometimes we must fight to find hope, but it is our greatest comfort and our greatest weapon.

Questions for the reader to consider

1. Who and what do you care about? What are your top skills and gifts?
2. Have you found your sacred purpose?
3. Do you – or could you – look for hope?

Glossary

ADHD – attention deficit hyperactivity disorder

Anti-racist – a person who opposes racism and promotes racial tolerance

ASD – autism spectrum disorder (sometimes referred to as autistic spectrum condition)

CAMHS – child and adolescent mental health services

Cisgendered – the gender of the person is the same as was assigned at birth

CPV – child-to-parent violence (sometimes referred to as APV – adolescent-to-parent violence)

DMDD – disruptive mood dysregulation disorder

Dyscalculia – difficulty in understanding numbers

Dyslexia – difficulty in understanding words

Dyspraxia – difficulty with motor skills (large and small)

EHCP – education, health and care plan

Gender fluid – when a person's gender identity is not fixed

Gender identity – an individual's personal sense of having a particular gender

Intersectional – initially being both female and of colour, now widened to other areas of marginalisation

Managed move – a move from one school to another where the child is still given access to teaching in the meantime, between schools

Masking – actions autistic people make to fit in, by blending in with those around them, even at the cost of their mental health

Non-binary – standing outside of binary genders associated with male or female

NVR – non-violent resistance, a strategy begun by Haim Omer to help people through conflict

PDA – pathological demand avoidance: demand avoidance outside of the range of what is considered to be normal

P-Ex – permanent exclusion

Queer – an umbrella term for people who are not heterosexual or cisgender

Section 20 – where a child is put back into the care of the local authority but with overall control remaining with the parents

SENCo – the special needs co-ordinator in a school

Sexuality – a person's identity in relation to the gender or genders to which they are typically attracted; sexual orientation

Transgender – (trans) someone whose gender identity or gender expression does not correspond with their sex assigned at birth

USEFUL RESOURCES

Books on Race

Brit(ish) – Afua Hirsch
How to Be an Antiracist – Ibram X. Kendi
So You Want to Talk About Race – Ijeoma Oluo
Talking to Children About Race – Loretta Andrews and Ruth Hill
White Fragility – Robin Diangelo

Charities

ADHD Foundation (https://www.adhdfoundation.org.uk)
Adoption UK (https://www.adoptionuk.org)
British Dyslexia Association (https://www.bdadyslexia.org.uk/dyscalculia)
Corum – Family and Childcare (https://www.familyandchildcaretrust.org)
Dyscalculia Association (http://www.dyscalculiaassociation.uk)
Dyspraxia Foundation (https://dyspraxiafoundation.org.uk)
Local Offer – tells you what's on offer locally for your

children with SEND. Found on your local authority website under the page 'Local Offer'.

MENCAP – for people with disability, including learning disability (https://www.mencap.org.uk)

Mermaids – helps gender-diverse young people and their families (https://mermaidsuk.org.uk)

National Autistic Society (https://www.autism.org.uk)

National Network of Parent Carer Forums (https://nnpcf.org.uk)

PDA – for help with pathological demand avoidance (https://www.pdasociety.org.uk)

Stonewall – LGBTQIA+ support and campaigns (https://www.stonewall.org.uk)

Facebook Groups

ADHD Warrior Squad (https://www.facebook.com/groups/317336065275307)

Black-owned Economy (https://www.facebook.com/groups/249229526309790)

EHCP Professional Parents (https://www.facebook.com/groups/270270486771556)

It's Not Just You (https://www.facebook.com/groups/itsnotjustyou)

Not Fine in School (https://www.facebook.com/groups/NFISFamilySupport)

Parenting Mental Health (https://www.facebook.com/groups/parentingmentalhealth)

SEND National Crisis (https://www.facebook.com/groups/190343344893926)

Mental Health

Beyond Charity (https://wearebeyond.org.uk)
MIND (https://www.mind.org.uk)
Samaritans (https://www.samaritans.org)
YoungMinds (https://www.youngminds.org.uk)

NOTES

1. Latham, S. (2017) *A White Guy Talks Race.* In Reddie, A. G., with Hudson Roberts, W. and Richards, G. (eds) *Journeying to Justice: Contributions to the Baptist Traditions Across the Black Atlantic.* Milton Keynes: Paternoster Press, p. 84.
2. Shafak, E. (2022) *The Island of Missing Trees.* London: Penguin Books Ltd.
3. Art Therapies for Children. Available at: https://www.artstherapies.org.uk (accessed 13 July 2022).
4. NHS Digital. (2021) 'Mental Health of Children and Young People in England 2021'. Available at: https://digital.nhs.uk/data-and-information/publications/statistical/mental-health-of-children-and-young-people-in-england/2021-follow-up-to-the-2017-survey (accessed 13 July 2022).
5. NHS Digital. (2018) 'Mental Health of Children and Young People in England, 2017'. Available at https://digital.nhs.uk/data-and-information/publications/statistical/mental-health-of-children-and-young-people-in-england/2017/2017 (accessed 13 July 2022).
6. YoungMinds. (2021) 'The Impact of Covid-19 on Young People with Mental Health Needs'. Available at: https://www.youngminds.org.uk/about-us/reports-and-impact/coronavirus-impact-on-young-people-with-mental-health-needs/ (accessed 13 July 2022)
7. Correspondence from Claire Murdoch and Professor Tim Kendall to Rt Hon. Jeremy Hunt MP. (17 August 2021). Available at: https://publications.parliament.uk/pa/cm5802/cmselect/cmhealth/17/report.html
8. Russell, G., Stapley, S., Newlove-Delgado, T., Salmon, A., White, R., Warren, F., Pearson, A., Ford, T. (2021) 'Time

trends in autism diagnosis over 20 years: a UK population-based cohort study'. *Journal of Child Psychology and Psychiatry*, 63(6), pp. 674–689.

9. Low, K. (2020) '20 Signs and Symptoms of ADHD in Girls'. Available at https://www.verywellmind.com/adhd-in-girls-symptoms-of-adhd-in-girls-20547 (accessed 4 July 2022).
10. Strand, S., Lindorff, A. (2020) 'Ethnic Disproportionality in the Identification of High-Incidence Special Educational Needs: A National Longitudinal Study Ages 5 to 11'. *Exceptional Children*, 87(3), pp.344–368.
11. NHS Digital. (2022) 'Autism Statistics, April 2021 to March 2022'. Available at: https://digital.nhs.uk/data-and-information/publications/statistical/autism-statistics/april-2021-to-march-2022 (accessed 23 June 2022).
12. National Autistic Society. 'What is Autism?'. Available at https://www.autism.org.uk/advice-and-guidance/what-is-autism (accessed 4 July 2022)
13. Tirraora, T. (2019) 'SEND Children are being "traumatised" by not getting the help they need in schools'. Available at: https://www.specialneedsjungle.com/send-children-being-traumatised-by-not-getting-help-need-schools/ (accessed 23 June 2022).
14. YoungMinds. (2019) *YoungMinds Impact Report 2018–2019.* Available at: https://www.youngminds.org.uk/media/o25lazbr/youngminds-impact-report-2018-19.pdf (accessed 4 April 2022).
15. Kessler, R., Berglund, P., Demler, O., Jin, R., Merikangas, K. R., & Walters, E. E. (2005) 'Lifetime prevalence and age-of-onset distributions of DSM-IV disorders in the National Comorbidity Survey Replication'. *Archives of General Psychiatry*, 62(6), pp. 593–602.
16. Grant, C. (2021) Tweet from @CarrieGrant1 on 9 September 2021. Available at: https://twitter.com/CarrieGrant1/status/1413395330012418048 (accessed 4 April 2022).
17. Racine, N., MacArthur, B. A., Cooke, J., Eirich, R., Zhu, J., Madigan, S. (2017) 'Global Prevalence of Depressive and Anxiety Symptoms in Children and Adolescents During COVID-19: A Meta-analysis'. *JAMA Pediatrics*, 175(11), pp. 1142–1150.
18. NHS England. (2016) 'The NHS Five Year Forward View for Mental Health'. Available at: https://www.england.nhs.uk/publication/the-five-year-forward-view-for-mental-health/

19. The figures were worked out in a slightly different way year to year, but we do know that the increase in referrals for the year 19/20 was 35 per cent, and the increase in those being seen was 4 per cent. Lennon, M. (2021) 'The State of Children's Mental Health Services 2020/21'. Available at: https://www.childrens-commissioner.gov.uk/report/mental-health-services-2019-20.
20. Andrews, D. et al. (2022) 'Amygdala Changes in Individuals with Autism Linked to Anxiety'. Available at: https://www.sciencedaily.com/releases/2022/02/220210154235.htm (accessed 20 June 2022).
21. Tajima-Pozo, K., Yus, M., Ruiz-Manrique, G., Lewczuk, A., Arrazola, J., Montanes-Rada, F. (2016) 'Amygdala Abnormalities in Adults with ADHD'. *Journal of Attention Disorders*, 22(7), pp. 671–678.
22. American Psychiatric Association. (2013) *Diagnostic and Statistical Manual for Mental Disorders*. Washington: American Psychiatric Association Publishing.
23. Wing, L., Gould, J. (2022) 'Diagnostic Interview for Social and Communication Disorders'. Available at: https://www.autism.org.uk/what-we-do/diagnosticservices/disco
24. NHS. 'Symptoms of Dyslexia'. Available at: https://www.nhs.uk/conditions/dyslexia/symptoms/ (accessed 5 July 2022).
25. The Dyslexia Association. Available at: https://www.dyslexia.uk.net
26. The Dyslexia Association. 'Symptoms of Dyscalculia'. Available at: https://www.dyslexia.uk.net/specific-learning-difficulties/dyscalculia/the-signs-of-dyscalculia/ (accessed 5 July 2022).
27. NHS. 'Symptoms of Dyspraxia'. Available at: https://www.nhs.uk/conditions/developmental-coordination-disorder-dyspraxia/symptoms/ (accessed 6 July 2022).
28. The Bible. Proverbs, 22:6. New International Version (2011). London: Hodder and Stoughton.
29. Warrier, V., Greenberg, D.M., Weir, E., Buckingham, C., Smith, P., Meng-Chuan, M., Allison, C. & Baron-Cohen, S. (2020) 'Elevated rates of autism, other neurodevelopmental and psychiatric diagnoses, and autistic traits in transgender and gender-diverse individuals'. *Nature Communications*, 11, 3959.
30. Bradlow, J., Bartram, F., Guasp, A., & Jadva, V. (2017) *School Report: The experiences of lesbian, gay, bi and trans young people in Britain's schools in 2017*. Available at: https://www.stonewall.

org.uk/system/files/the_school_report_2017.pdf (accessed 4 April 2022).

31. Stonewall. 'The Truth About Trans'. Available at: https://www.stonewall.org.uk/truth-about-trans (accessed 14 June 2022).
32. Mermaids. Available at: https://mermaidsuk.org.uk
33. CQC. 'Tavistock and Portman NHS Foundation Trust – Gender Identity' (report updated 20 January 2021. Available at: https://www.cqc.org.uk/provider/RNK/inspection-summary#genderis (accessed 15 June 2022).
34. The Cass Review. (2022) 'Independent review of gender identity services for children and young people: Interim report'. Available at: https://cass.independent-review.uk/wp-content/uploads/2022/03/Cass-Review-Interim-Report-Final-Web-Accessible.pdf (accessed 15 June 2022).
35. Fisk, Knudson, De Cuypere, & Bockting (1974), 2010b Retrieved 4th July 22 from: https://www.england.nhs.uk/wp-content/uploads/2017/04/gender-development-service-children-adolescents.pdf
36. Ainsworth, C. (2015) 'Sex redefined'. *Nature*, 518, pp. 288–291.
37. Fausto-Sterling, Anne. (2000) *Sexing the Body: Gender Politics and the Construction of Sexuality*. New York: Basic Books.
38. Sax, L. (2002) 'How Common Is Intersex? A Response to Anne Fausto-Sterling'. *Journal of Sex Research*, 39 (3), pp. 174–178.
39. Crenshaw, K. (1989) 'Demarginalizing the Intersection of Race and Sex: A Black Feminist Critique of Antidiscrimination Doctrine, Feminist Theory and Antiracist Politics'. Available at: https://philpapers.org/archive/CREDTI.pdf?ncid=txtlnkus-aolp00000603 (accessed 16 June 2022).
40. *Oxford English Dictionary*. (1989) Oxford: Oxford University Press.
41. Mustafa, T. (2022) 'Nearly half of black people believe hair discrimination has increased in recent years, says research'. *Metro*. Available at: https://metro.co.uk/2022/08/15/around-46-of-black-people-believe-hair-discrimination-has-increased-17183584/ (accessed 29 September 2022).
42. Millman, D. (2010) *Way of the Peaceful Warrior: A book that changes lives*. New York: Peaceful Warrior ePublishing.
43. Valdez-Symonds, S. (2018) '70 Years After Windrush', Amnesty International UK. Available at: https://www.amnesty.org.uk/blogs/yes-minister-it-human-rights-issue/seventy-years-after-windrush?utm_source=google&utm_medium=grant&utm_

campaign=AWA_HRUK_windrush&utm_content=windrush%20scandal%20explained (accessed 7 July 2022).

44. Kirkup, R. and Winnett, R. (2012) 'Theresa May interview: We're going to give immigrants a really hostile reception', the *Telegraph*.
45. McIntosh, P. (1988). 'White Privilege: Unpacking the Invisible Knapsack'. Available at: https://psychology.umbc.edu/wp-content/uploads/sites/57/2016/10/White-Privilege_McIntosh-1989.pdf (accessed 22 September 2022).
46. *Oxford English Dictionary*. (1989) Oxford: Oxford University Press.
47. Omer, H. (2004) *Non-Violent Resistance: A New Approach to Violent and Self-destructive Children*. Cambridge: Cambridge University Press.
48. Attwood, T., Moller Nielsen, A., Callesen, K. (2009) *CAT Kit (Cognitive Affective Training)*. Arlington: Future Horizons.
49. National Autistic Society. 'Pathological Demand Avoidance'. Available at https://www.autism.org.uk/advice-and-guidance/topics/diagnosis/pda/parents-and-carers (accessed 6 July 2022).
50. Alia-Klein, N., Goldstein, R. Z., Tomasi, D., Zhang, L., Fagin-Jones, S., Telang, F., Wang, G.-J., Fowler, J. S., & Volkow, N. D. (2007) 'What's in a word? No versus Yes differentially engage the lateral orbitofrontal cortex'. *Emotion*, 7(3), pp.649–659.
51. De Montfort University. (2019) 'Research shows praising children five times a day has positive impact'. Available at: https://www.dmu.ac.uk/about-dmu/news/2019/october/research-shows-praising-children-five-times-a-day-has-positive-impact.aspx (accessed 8 July 2022).
52. Westwood, S. et al. (2019) 'Five Praises a Day Tips'. Available at: https://www.dmu.ac.uk/documents/about-dmu-documents/news/tips-for-using-praise.pdf (accessed 8 July 2022).
53. NHS. 'Overview: Cognitive behavioural therapy'. Available at: https://www.nhs.uk/mental-health/talking-therapies-medicine-treatments/talking-therapies-and-counselling/cognitive-behavioural-therapy-cbt/overview/ (accessed 20 September 2022).
54. Priory. 'Dialectical behaviour therapy (DBT): What it is, how it works and who can use it'. Available at: https://www.priorygroup.com/blog/dialectical-behaviour-therapy-dbt (accessed 20 September 2022).
55. Joseph, S., Regel, S., Harris, B. and Murphy, D. (2017) 'What

to expect when being counselled for trauma and post-traumatic stress disorder'. Available at: https://www.bacp.co.uk/about-therapy/trauma-and-ptsd/ (accessed 20 September 2022).

56. Shapiro, F. (2001) *EMDR: The Breakthrough 'Eye Movement' Therapy for Overcoming Anxiety, Stress, and Trauma*. LaVergne, USA: Ingram Publisher Services.
57. Porteous-Sebhouhian, B. (2022) 'What is somatic therapy and why is it perfect for trauma recovering?'. Available at: https://www.mentalhealthtoday.co.uk/blog/therapy/what-is-somatic-therapy-and-why-is-it-perfect-for-trauma-recovery (accessed 20 September 2022).
58. The Theraplay Institute. 'What is Theraplay?'. Available at: https://theraplay.org/what-is-theraplay/ (accessed 20 September 2022).
59. England – National Association of Parent Carer Forums, https://nnpcf.org.uk. Scotland – National Parent Forum of Scotland, https://www.npfs.org.uk. Wales – https://www.allwalesforum.org.uk. Northern Ireland – https://www.facebook.com/CarersNI/.
60. Personal communication via email (5 July 2016, 15.29).
61. Ashmall, L., Cacciottolo, M. (2017) 'I Sent My Adopted Son Back Into Care'. Available at: https://www.bbc.co.uk/news/uk-38764302 (4 July 2022).
62. Puffett, N. (2018) 'Investigation Reveals Increase In Adoption Placement Breakdowns'. Available at: https://www.cypnow.co.uk/features/article/investigation-reveals-increase-in-adoption-placement-breakdowns (accessed 4 July 2022).
63. Thorley, W., Coates, A. (2017) 'Child–Parent Violence (CPV): exploratory exercise Impact on parent/carers when living with CPV'. Available at: https://www.academia.edu/31433287/Child_-Parent_Violence_CPV_exploratory_exercise_Impact_on_parent_carers_when_living_with_CPV (accessed 15 July 2022).
64. You Magazine. (2020) 'When Adoption Fails: The Guilt of Giving a Child Back'. Available at: https://www.you.co.uk/adoption-breakdown-when-adoption-fails/ (accessed 4 July 2022).
65. The Week. (2017) 'Why half of UK adoptive families are struggling with violence'. Available at: https://www.theweek.co.uk/88631/why-half-of-uk-adoptive-families-are-struggling-with-violence (accessed 4 July 2022).

66. Long, J. (2019) 'Two-thirds of adoptive parents experience violence or aggression from their child'. Available at: https://www.channel4.com/news/two-thirds-of-adoptive-parents-experience-violence-or-aggression-from-their-child (accessed 4 July 2022).
67. National Institute of Mental Health. (2017) 'Disruptive Mood Dysregulation Disorder: Overview'. Available at: https://www.nimh.nih.gov/health/topics/disruptive-mood-dysregulation-disorder-dmdd/disruptive-mood-dysregulation-disorder (accessed 4 July 2022).
68. UK Government. (2022) 'Adoption Support Fund (ASF)'. Available at: https://www.gov.uk/guidance/adoption-support-fund-asf (accessed 4 July 2022).
69. Children Act 1989, Section 20. (2016) Available at: https://www.legislation.gov.uk/ukpga/1989/41/section/20 (accessed 4 July 2022).
70. Albiston, K. (2016) 'Domestic Homicide Review into the Death of "Sarah"/2016'. Available at: https://www.northumberland.gov.uk/NorthumberlandCountyCouncil/media/Safer-Northumberland-docs/DHR-Executive-Summary-Sarah.pdf (accessed 4 July 2022).
71. Hughes, D., Baylin, J. (2012) *Brain-Based Parenting: The Neuroscience of Caregiving for Healthy Attachment*. New York: WW Norton & Co.
72. The Child Psychology Service. 'Blocked Care'. Available at: https://thechildpsychologyservice.co.uk/advice-strategy/blocked-care/ (accessed 24 September 2022).
73. Ritter, W. (2016) *Beastly Bones*. New York: Workman Publishing Company.
74. Donath, O. (2017) *Regretting Motherhood*. Berkeley: North Atlantic Books.
75. Tweet from @crowsfault on 10 March 2022. Available at: https://twitter.com/crowsfault/status/1502001835779014666?lang=en-GB

Acknowledgements

Our primary thanks go to our children – you have motivated us to be the ever-evolving parents you need. In so doing, you have moved us towards becoming more than we knew we could be. And for all the times during the writing of this book when we said, 'Sure, dinner will be in a minute . . .'

Thanks to our late mummas – fierce women who loved and believed in us.

Thanks to our 'village' – those who have faithfully walked alongside us, cheerleading us and never judging. Special thanks to: Our Space Family, Luke and Hugo, Morag, Dr Mala D. German, Lisa Camilerri, Lime Pictures, The Autism and Girls Forum and those who taught us about Trauma Therapy and NVR. Very special thanks to our Autism Family Support Group – thank you for holding the space for us, for 'getting' us, and for your loyalty.

Big thanks to our publishing agent, Charlie Brotherstone, who got it from the start and was the first to show an interest. The title was yours.

Our publishers: thanks to Jillian Young, who believed this book needed to be written and has been a constant source of encouragement; to Jillian Stewart, who has kept us on track to print; and to Matthew Crossey, who has enthusiastically championed this book to market.

And, finally, thanks to all those represented in the communities this book is about. Your stories matter, your voices matter. We see you, we hear you.

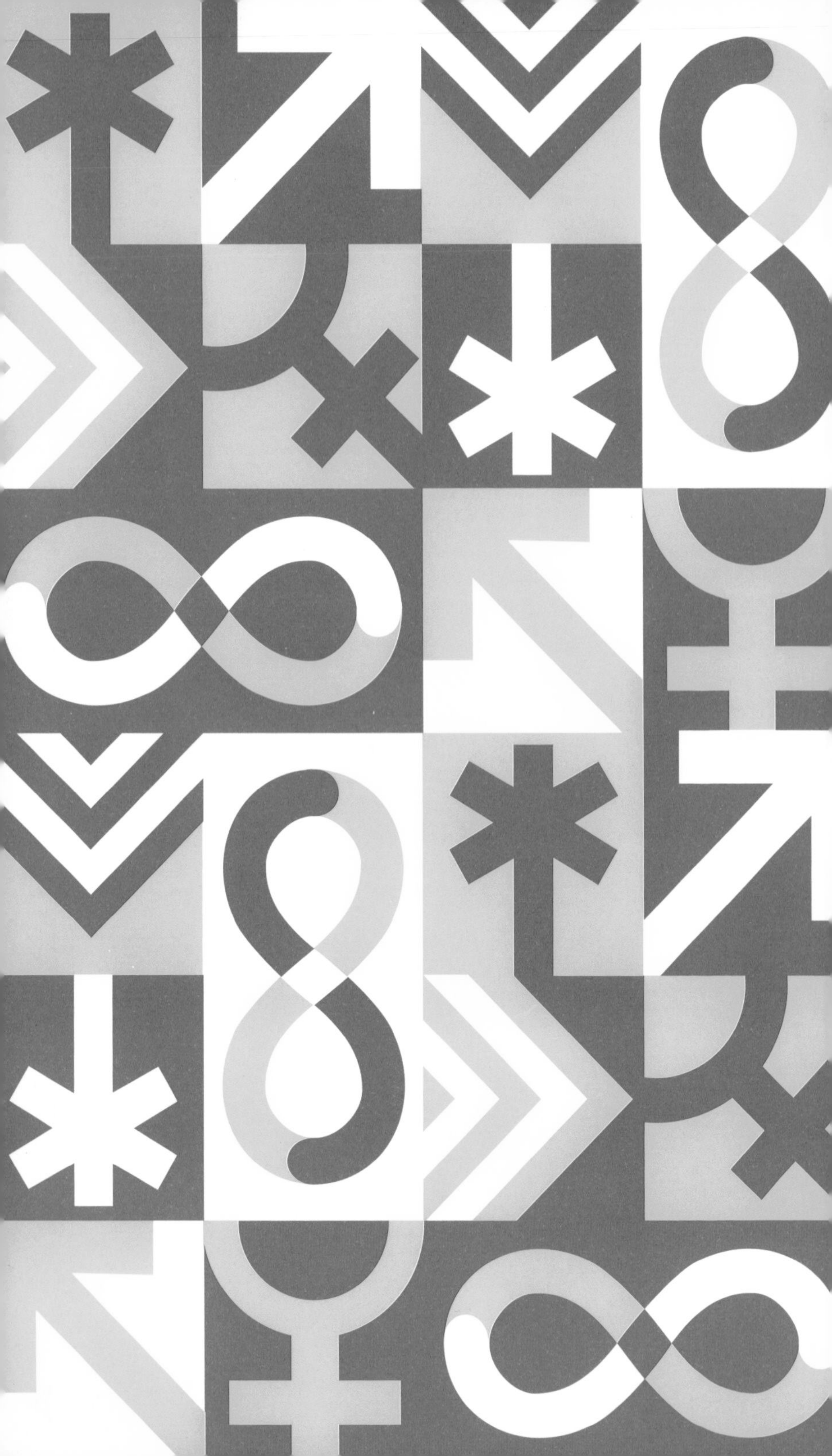